BODY LOVE

A new, gentle, simple art of movement that results in the physical, mental and emotional harmony that is total well-being.

BODY LOVE

Movement for Total Well-Being

Peggy Brusseau

THORSONS PUBLISHING GROUP
Wellingborough, Northamptonshire
———— · ————
Rochester, Vermont

First published 1987

British Library Cataloguing in Publication Data

Brusseau, Peggy
Body love: movement for total well-being.
1. Exercise   2. Physical fitness
I. Title
613.7′1   RA781

ISBN 0-7225-1437-9

Printed and bound in Great Britain.

Dedication

For everyone who has a body . . . and desires that joy, wellness and progress be possible through it.

Acknowledgements

My thanks to the hundreds of men, women and children who have attended my classes over the years. Their moving, laughing and questioning contribution has been both essential and exciting to my work.

My love and gratitude to Carolyn Baxter and Kurt Weithaler who not only modelled for the illustrations throughout this book, but have been dear and loyal friends to me and my work over many years.

And very special thanks to Peter for his enduring trust.

Contents

Chapter 1
You can do it!

Why are you unhappy with your body?

I bet you're surprised that I should ask you such a question. Even though I don't know you, I know that you don't like your body *as it is*, I know that the last time you felt really good about your body was ages ago. I know that for the first four or five years of your life you had unlimited and uninhibited pride in your body. You spent those years becoming familiar with the way your body worked. You explored the range of movements available to you. Everything was new and exciting. I know that you lived every experience through your body.

Do you remember?

During your early years everything seemed possible. You felt physical exuberance, delight in your body, and an uncensored quality of joy in all that you did. I know that that very quality is your birthright. You were given your body, born into it with an awareness that it is yours for the duration. Yours as a lifeline to experience, sensation, intimacy, creation and communication.

Your young body was a celebration of life. What about now? Do you find that:

- It's difficult to concentrate, to get interested in things. Your senses sometimes close down so much that very little sensation or excitement can get in, or out. You feel dull, monotonous, bored (you never felt bored when you were four years old). Other people pick this up, they sense your weariness. It's infectious and it's called **lethargy.**
- You don't like being looked at as you move, especially if you are doing new or unusual things like dancing, playing a game with your kids, wearing new clothes or shoes. You feel very frustrated with your body at times. Why can't you control it more? Why doesn't it seem to fit in with

your personality? How did you ever get to feel this way? Is it really *your* body? This feeling is **awkwardness.**

- When in the presence of a powerful, more self-assured person, you unconsciously begin to mimic their actions, their posture, their demeanour. Your own personality, your whole being, seems swamped by their more dynamic and purposeful personality. You find yourself agreeing with them, doing what *they* want and only later regretting that you couldn't have been more assertive yourself. This distressing syndrome is very common. It is **de-personalization.**
- If you relax at all, it's in a superficial, preoccupied way. You probably don't sleep soundly. Your 'action' switch is stuck in the 'on' position. You respond to everything, no matter how trivial or important, with the same amount of energy. Maybe you feel important behaving in this way, maybe others find it impressive. You may receive praise and hear people comment with incredulity: 'what a tireless worker! So much energy and buzz'. Only you know how much you *really* get done. When your body isn't trying to cope with this 'all-or-nothing' taskmaster, it's desperately trying to recover. So when you go home you collapse in a heap or feel completely wiped out. This pattern of behaviour is called '**hyperbusyness'.**

We have established two very important facts. Firstly, that there was a time in your life years ago when you felt a wonderful ease and delight in your body. A time when all of life seemed within your grasp. Secondly, that your life today contains elements of the kind of unhappiness and dis-ease just mentioned. So I will repeat my question: Why are you unhappy with your body?

How did this unhappiness come about?

Your delight, your sense of possession, your ease with your body that you had as a young child diminished as the process of becoming social took hold. As you became more and more channelled in your activities, as your outlook and attitudes narrowed, you began to *use* your body, rather than to *be* it.

Your body wants to be a reflection of you, it wants to respond to your thoughts and feelings, it wants to express them and be part of them, it wants to be well. But your body can be none of these if you just use it, because a used body is a distant body. It is no longer connected with you and so it stops responding with the same directness that it once did. It becomes 'unwell' — perhaps not in any profound or even obvious sense at first, but when your body becomes isolated from you it quite simply loses its way. It becomes a shell that you carry around everywhere. No wonder you become unhappy with it.

Your body does try to warn you. It signals distance and isolation so that you will stop and remedy the problem. Your body never considers that you might just keep on behaving in a way that ignores it. It cannot believe the harsh tactics used to silence or shun its signals: drugs, over-eating, over-work, lack of laughter and touch. Where did you learn that?

But you aren't the only person who uses your body. Your aches and pains and sags and worries have become big business.

Everyone knows that '36-24-36' is a perfect combination; if you aren't 'tall, dark and handsome . . .' don't apply; of course, 'blondes have more fun'; here, 'this'll put hairs on your chest' and so on. You can begin to feel that you are never good enough. Big business uses your body to sell you and I that message and we believe it!

You probably received one of these suggestions within the last day:

- *Big Business (Food)*: sells us diets and real things; ultimate experiences and goodness; power breakfasts and sexy chocolate bars.
- *Big Business (Fashion)*: sells us slimness and sleekness; long legs; confident casuals; powerful business suits and ever-changing styles.
- *Big Business (Bodies)*: sells us the average age of 25; brilliant white teeth, rigorous games, bulging muscles, gorgeous hair, flawless skin.
- *Big Business (Health)*: sells us aches and pains, depression and heartburn; colds and flu; lots and lots of medicine to cure it all.

Recently a new branch has been added to the conglomerate:

- *Big Business (Fitness)*: sells us a package called fitness training.

This is a really profitable branch of Big Business because anyone who buys this package is a sure bet for all of the other packages mentioned above. Big Business (Fitness) promises:

- *Females*: now you *too* can have big breasts, a small waist, sleek thighs and long legs, a flat stomach, tight buttocks, white teeth and thin but strong arms.
- *Males*: all of *this* can be yours — huge biceps, broad shoulders, narrow waist and hips, massive thighs, white teeth and irresistable charm.

There are several ways of receiving this package. You can buy records, tapes, videos, or you can attend a class. In each case, you will probably put yourself through pain — to the accompaniment of beaty music. Somehow, you will *want* to feel this pain. You will probably have purchased a bright stretchy leotard, supplied by Big Business (Fashion). If you attend a class, then you will be lined up in straight rows with many other people and shouted at by a person — the teacher. You will imitate this person and somehow you won't mind if he or she comes round to check that you are feeling liberal amounts of pain in the right places. When the class is finished, you will enrol for another ten or twenty, even though your ankle is sprained, your varicose veins are throbbing, your back is in agony and you still haven't caught your breath. At least, you think to yourself, you'll be fit.

Although you don't mean to be predictable, a part of you really wants the package. You want to look and feel great. You want to live up to those ideals and stereotypes. Even though the cost is so enormously high you still want to 'go for it' with gusto.

You probably recognize a physical condition that could, in part, belong to you. You recognize beauty, even if it is manufactured or painted on. Like, in this case, attracts like: the beauty within you is roused by the beauty you see and aspire to. There is nothing wrong in that, but what a pity that the way you try to be beautiful is so ugly.

And why try so hard for Big Business? It doesn't matter to them whether you are young or old, shapely or flabby, fit or breathless, large or small. They will promise you all of their best-selling features in any case — it's not *their* problem if you aren't able to conform to the outline. Big Business doesn't acknowledge physical variety or handicap or healthy, joyful, active ways of ageing. It doesn't care whether you are well and happy. Big Business wants you to strive to fill their manufactured image.

If you have distanced yourself from your body, and if you have allowed that distance to broaden, then you are almost certain to get ill. In the early days, before the distance and isolation is profound, your illness will be pseudo-illness. Does one of these describe your symptoms?

- You don't remember when they started or what caused them, but they are persistant or recurring and feel most uncomfortable during your leisure time. They may be mild or nearly unbearable and may occur anywhere in your body. They are **aches and pains.**
- You may feel overwhelmed by this at times, but it mostly remains nagging in the background. This symptom explains a lot that is poor or mediocre about your work, your health, and your general outlook. Even so, you don't really know the cause of your **fatigue.**
- You usually suffer this in one area of your body. It recurs with monotonous regularity, but, even so, you are always surprised by it. **Stiffness and tension** will prevent you from doing some tasks but, amazingly, not other activities that you may enjoy a little bit more.
- These symptoms may appear as early as 25 years old and include sagging muscles, poor posture and general loss of mobility. The symptoms are worse after meals or just before going to work. Any of the other pseudo-illnesses may be **age-induced** problems too.
- After you have endured a whole series of 'preliminary' symptoms your ailment becomes quite debilitating and may then recur throughout your life. Often the first indication of the presence of **digestive, circulatory or respiratory ailments** occurs at an unhappy or worrying time for you.
- If you are middle aged then you may be familiar with this affliction. It is most obvious in the evenings and at weekends or holidays. Your **loss of stamina** usually improves when you stop challenging your body to new and varied activities.
- This feeling comes over you suddenly and without warning. You may feel fine one moment and the next feel quite low or irritable. You can quickly shift **moodiness** by making yourself do something.
- Do you sometimes feel flushed, sweaty and perhaps nauseated? Or do you feel just slightly

uncomfortable all of the time? Do you experience loss of concentration or come out with inane chatter, stuttering or clumbsiness? This ailment is **nervousness.**
- Are you quite certain that you are fully capable of handling the situation? Do muteness, respiratory constriction and the urge to run occur in chronic waves, without remission, at the thought of it? Or do you experience **lack of confidence** as a severe but brief moment of disquiet?
- Your brain may be unwilling to respond to any of the challenges of daily life. In particular, those relating to work, study, home maintenance, news broadcasts or financial bookkeeping. **Mental dullness** may leave you appearing normal in other ways.

Somehow these symptoms can appear without you noticing. Their effects can be so gradual that you do not attribute them to anything insidious. And in a way, how could you? They are all of your own making. They are the patterns and habits of ill health that you have established instead of getting to really know your body again. And we project this to others:

'How are you?'
'Oh, not too bad.'

'Are you all right?'
'As well as can be expected.'

'How are you doing?'
'Could be worse.'

How depressing.

You don't remember choosing to feel unwell or distant from your body but, in fact, you *have* chosen distance and ill health. Maybe you stopped believing in your body, in its needs and expressions, because you were sold on someone else's idea of how you should be.

No wonder your body malfunctions. No wonder it sort of tags along, all droopy and reluctant. It probably has a bad case of 'nobody loves me'.

You may not feel ill at present, but do you feel good? Do you feel really good? Do you feel great?

Later in life your body may get into really deep trouble. Pseudo-illness may move over for the real thing. Your body might just stop wanting to try for you. It may lose its motivation, its drive, its will to live. Do you want that to happen to you?

Your body's real purpose, that of providing you with arms and eyes and excitement for the life you live through — is denied when you remain ignorant of its real needs. All of those little complaints and warning signals can become deep-seated and cause severe health problems. Your body can create real illness. It will try finally and desperately to communicate with you before devising a worthy form of self-destruction to complete its isolation. What a sad, desolate ending to such a beautiful beginning.

You started your life in support of your body. You needed and wanted it. Your personality was bound joyously and inextricably to your body, but things may well have changed. Since those early days, you may have 'unplugged' some connections.

Your most vulnerable connection is that which unites your outer self with your inner self. It is formed entirely from communication and is the connection most brutalized by current life-style patterns.

Your hand is very different from your shoulder but would you like to be without the arm that stretches between them? You know that then, of course, your hand would no longer work, so you tend to take care of your arm, hand and shoulder.

Your body is very different from your thoughts and feelings but would you like to be without the communication that connects them? Looking after the connection just a little bit is not enough because poor connections mean 'poor' living. A disconnected body *is* yours but you are left very aloof from it. It is tenacious, always with you, yet you are isolated from it. It is a burden, an imposition, a necessity. You may resent it and want it and be ignorant of it all at once. But it needn't be so.

You can take possession of your body again.

It doesn't matter what size, shape, age, or type of physique you are. You can stop using your body, stop distancing yourself from it, stop being ill in it. Instead, you can *be* your body and from that moment your whole life may change and improve.

You have a second chance to be happy with your body. To feel joy and exuberance through it. To be delighted with yourself. It's all up to you.

A body that is yours is truly you. It is well and full of vitality; it responds to mental, emotional and physical signals; it extends itself to challenges and change; it becomes fully aware of you and allows that awareness to affect your behaviour, your habits, your life.

A body that has secure links with you creates opportunities for all aspects of your character to work together. You create quality in your life, become a strong, unified personality.

The question is, how?

Movement Design is a new, gentle art of movement. It teaches a collection of simple movements, the practice of which sparks off a wonderful chain of events within you. Events that result in the physical, mental and emotional harmony that is your birthright.

Movement is a direct route to each person, to the you inside your body. Movement encourages your body to rebuild and strengthen its links with you.

You are made up of body, mind and emotion but you may well have left your body out of things lately. Unless you become your body, re-connect with it, you may remain in a narrow, unhealthy, and probably unhappy state. But when you unify, become a team, a network, a mutual admiration society within your whole personality, nothing will stop you from experiencing *real* health.

Here is what you need:
- A real willingness to make the changes that will reinstate the connections between your body and you
- A strong desire to experience vitality, calm, health, confidence, joy
- A belief in the ability of your body to gain or re-gain some degree of mobility, suppleness, strength, gracefulness, stamina and pride
- A sense of humour
- A desire to have fun
- A willingness to move — no matter how immobile you are or think you are — to the best of your ability

Here is what you get:
- Strong, positive self-images about you and your body
- Real health, mental acuity, poise and joyfulness
- Ease, both personal and physical, in most situations
- A growing awareness of yourself — your talents, abilities, characteristics, needs and ambitions
- Pleasure
- Numerous and frequent opportunities for laughter
- Strength, suppleness, grace, balance, stamina, pride and vitality
- Delight in your own ability to move
- The challenge and rewards of exploring your own personal potentials

And that's just the beginning. You can have as much fun as you like for as long as you like. You won't need to time yourself, push yourself or lock yourself away in a quiet room.

All you have to do is start.

Chapter 2

How to design your perfect body

A brief history of the body
The flower that couldn't blossom

Your body is the history of all bodies. Its movements, postures and physical attributes are a culmination of human living, moving and surviving over many thousands of years.

Your body is an inheritance. You receive it because of investments laid down generations ago.

Imagine humankind as a plant that is slowly establishing itself and creating its own suitable soil. Each new generation of seedlings has a slightly stronger chance of survival: a greater height and span of leaf, a firmer grip in the soil. In a similar way, you and I have benefited from the human lives before us.

You are born into an environment, full of other people, where most of what you do has been done before. Most of your natural enemies are known, most of your human traits and characteristics are already measured and validated. You have thousands of years of human error and success on which to base any choice or decision you might make.

Humankind has been successful in surviving a great many changes, most of them physical. To continue the analogy of the plant, humankind is weed-like: it has learned to take sustenance from even the most barren places, it is daring and also prolific. Humankind has become a vast acreage of leaf and branch and firm-rootedness; it has grown and spread and put out bud. But humankind has not blossomed.

In order for it to blossom, a number of things have to be right all at the same time. The plant, for instance, needs to be mature and have temperature, humidity and light in the correct measures. You have only three requirements, three essences that sustain you as an individual. These essences are your physical, your mental and your emotional selves. These are always with you and need only be present in the right proportions at the right time to enable you to blossom into your unique potential.

Your physical self holds power over these proportions, with your mental and emotional selves brought into the mix as your body determines. This is true for you, as an individual, and for culture. The moment of blossom — if it comes to you — is possible only if your body's needs are met because then and only then is there opportunity for mind and emotion to emerge in quantities sufficient for a state of balance within you — and ultimately within our culture.

The 'body' of culture is environment, climate, health, diet, housing. The 'mind' of culture is commerce, industry, farming, technology, ethics and mores. The 'emotion' of culture is art, religion, medicine, communications, education and family units. These three areas of need have not been in balance for long enough to enable *all* the individuals within the culture to gain their own, inner balance. This means that culture has survived in a 'juvenile' state for thousands of years and, just occasionally, each of its essential requirements have been met, but not all at once and never enough to pull the culture headlong out of immaturity into the full blossom of humanity that is its potential.

Your body is the history of all bodies, the reflection of all human progress and a legacy from all of those who went before you.

Here is their story. The story of your body so far.

Surviving

Humankind's very first challenge was survival and it was achieved by fulfilling the basic physical needs of life. Our mental and emotional selves were present, but in the very early period of human existence the body took the bulk of our attention and demanded an obvious priority over mind and emotion. There was a stark, daily reality of life versus death that confronted every human being and to ensure survival required constant bodily effort. Indeed, life *was* the body. The body was the indicator of life, the substance of life and the shape of life.

Survival was our occupation for a great many generations: a basic, day-to-day survival of which most of us have no current understanding. However, we do have a memory of, a bequest from, the humankind who lived to survive.

In all of the knowledge and understanding and experience that has patterned our existence, pain has been a constant motif. It has been with us through each phase of human development, has taken many guises and served many purposes. Our urge to survive was, in a way, the mother of pain: our bodies needed something between life and death, some voice to alert. Pain was a shout from the body. To this day, any person or culture pushed towards death will peel back the layers of history and precedent until this kernel of survival is reached. Here pain signals alarm. Here the battle of life versus death is fought. Here our struggle becomes the same as that of our predecessors.

Expression and emergence

Over the generations humankind gradually adapted — we are good at that. Where once we clung precariously to our environment, we began to control it. Once we were, like poppies, brief and scattered, then we were, like buttercups, taking hold.

We gained expertise in avoiding death by making tools, building shelters and outsmarting nasty animals. We remembered which plants we shouldn't eat and which were able to heal and sustain. We became more useful to one another by sharing effort and developing skills. We grew from being students to masters of our environment.

Ever so slightly, humankind began to raise its head, to gaze over a longer view. Life was just a little more definite, our bodies a little more likely to be there the next day. And as our confidence grew we began to celebrate our lives. We began using our bodies to give expression to life rather than simply contain it.

We mimed our fellows and learned to laugh. We played. We danced celebrations of season, birth, kinship and gender. We mimicked the animals. We demonstrated skills, competed with one another and taught our children to express fear, pain and anger through their movements.

Humankind was emerging. As our ability to survive gradually and definitely improved we formulated more powerful and secure images of ourselves. We knew our bodies, trusted them and acknowledged our reliance upon them and from that security we looked outwards and upwards. We compared our bodies to the other lifeforms around us and devised relationships. We saw ourselves relative to all else and that experience, that vision, was translated into bodily form. Our bodies then became the site of not just existence, but meaning.

The birth of ritual

Celebration and expression merged and compounded until our attitude towards our bodies became one of exultation and worship. We knew ourselves and our life only through our bodies and so every bodily action and function held great importance. To reinforce this importance, we created a formal median of physical experience. A formal structure for the relationships and sense of meaningfulness being gained through the body. This median was ritual. Ritual reiterated the patterns of life we perceived around us, it embodied them and led us to sculpt purpose and further meaning from our lives.

We no longer had to toil individually for survival — that became a group or tribal effort — and so our goals were extended beyond the day-to-day existence of individual bodily survival. We sought instead to communicate, to barter, to create definitions and establish similarities. All of these were goals pursued, initially, through the body — through dance, story-telling, competition, gesture — yet their pursuit was also the foundation of all art and belief, the foundation of all that enabled humankind to explore life through emotion and intellect.

In this era we were, like children, fascinated by ourselves. Every day was a confrontation with newness and variety. Just as children greet new things by touching and tasting, so humankind acquainted itself with new things by giving bodily attributes and characteristics to them. The body acted to absorb all experience and then distribute it between body, mind and emotion. In this way we discovered and exercised our mental and emotional anatomies. We broadened our lives, became broad-leaved and firm-rooted like thriving plants.

Throughout these changes, through every generation, the inheritance of pain remained. Pain is an individual sensation, it is solitary. In ritualizing our bodies and our movements, we created a bond between ourselves and others. We sparked kinship which, though not by any means eliminating or even diminishing pain, enabled people to cluster in empathy and understanding. We were able, due partly to pain, to become social and supportive groups: we were able to recognize in others what we felt in ourselves.

Our bodily experiences became our culture in those early days. Our rituals established patterns of self-worship that enabled us to share personal experience and self-image. What grew out of this collaboration was twofold.

On the one hand, we established firm cultural groups. These groupings undermined our sense of and perception of the individual just sufficiently to enable communication and communication allowed the exchange of common bodily experience and perception to shape a collective future and a social and cultural potential.

On the other hand, the pooling of individual experiences provided us with protection. By sharing our understanding we established a unified defence against the many factors able to prey on the human body: disease, attack, accident, famine, weather and season. All of these were made less terrifyingly powerful by the solidarity of the ritualized, cultured individual.

In the first instance, humankind made a precarious stretch into that which is not the body — that which is not the life of one person. In the second instance, all medical, artistic and religious frameworks were begun to preserve both the unique body and the group body.

This phase of our development saw our bodies become the source and the subject of ritual, saw pain become a shared experience, one which came closest, at that time, to shared or common emotion. We were childlike and full of excitement for our bodies — they were the form of our life and the bulk of its meaning. We were surviving, enduring, conquering, but also beginning to be emotional, mindful and social.

Symbol and analogy

Our bodily self-image grew ever stronger as we played

and challenged and explored. We were better able to care for the body, were more able to rely on it and enjoy it. And our successful lifestyle gave continuous reinforcement to our developing self-image so that we eventually became very proud creatures indeed.

We knew ourselves to be a part of all life, all our environment and we knew the world through its effects on our own bodies. Whereas previously we had celebrated ourselves through the formalities of ritual, now our enormous pride took us beyond ritual. In our efforts to explain the world and relate to it, we began to symbolize the body and make analogy with it. Any event or form or pattern obvious in the greater world was given a mirror in the smaller world of our bodies. Our sense of body became so acute that all of life was given a place and a meaning within us.

Perhaps at this moment in our history we were as close to blossom as we had ever been. We were successful survivors and quite probably happy. We were familiar with our environment and, more importantly, knew how to create an environment suited to our needs. We were emotional through our art and through our beliefs, and we were intellectual in our rapid establishment of towns, tools and agriculture. A strong and definite pattern of what was human had emerged. In the analogy of the plant, we were established.

However, the memory, the message, of survival still echoed in us. Woven in with our sense of belonging to life and our deep sense of physical meaning, was a barb of death, disease, and discomfort. Indigenous to our patch of ground was the blight of pain. No art or belief could rid us of it.

At this point, for the first time, we found discrepancy. Something poisoned what was otherwise becoming more beautiful, more meaningful, more powerful in us. Weren't we in every way a reflection of the world we knew? Didn't we celebrate and respond to every nuance of life? How could this thing still anchor us to what we used to be?

Our pride stepped beyond our bodies as we, again, compared ourselves to the life around us. And what we saw through our proud and advancing gaze made us begin, quite purposefully, to distance ourselves from it all.

Distance and schism

Our gaze landed most critically on animals and we decided that our close association with them must end. We no longer desired to recognize them as bodies with any likelihood of similitude to ours. We chose, instead, to believe ours the most perfect body, far better than any in the animal world, and we set about constructing a sturdy — in some ways impenetrable — barrier of difference and distance from them. We outlined the details of animal behaviour and forbade them in our rituals. We discouraged certain movements, postures and activities that implied any degree of animality in ourselves. We stopped treating animals with compassion or respect. Our culture slowly attempted to sever itself from the animal world and, as it did so, all of our attitudes, our rituals and our symbols altered or decayed.

Of course, to complete the separation was impossible. We slept, ate, eliminated, breathed and created as did animals. The basic functions of the body and our uses of it prevented the complete severence we sought.

For the first time we felt loss of power over our bodies. So we declared that, whilst having to endure these animal similarities, we at least had a spirit and, further, that our spirit could take flight, it could soar beyond this body, it needed none of this world. We even convinced ourselves that this spirit could feel no pain. That, at least, seemed to resolve the problem of our painful inheritance. Now we could put pain in its place alongside the animalness of our bodies. Or so we thought.

In effect, we abandoned our selves. We created a schism between our body and all that was within us. We grew to despise our resemblance to other life. We nurtured disdain towards our bodies because they seemed to bind us to an animal reality that we no longer found tolerable.

The plant, so close to blossom, grew brittle and acid: the seed-bed of our culture became soured.

Privacy, punishment and pain

From survival we had gestated through ritual, self-worship, and society. At this new juncture we fell into self-abnegation. We began to subdue our bodily expressions, deny basic bodily needs, decry our shape, our movements, our parts, our labours. We purported disgust for our bodies and declared them to be prisons of our spirit. What emerged were two social precepts opposing those of earlier humankind:

we sought physical privacy;
we sought to inflict punishment upon ourselves

Privacy renounced the body and made the body

embarrassed. Privacy said that what was functional and productive about our bodies was ugly and distasteful and should be hidden. At the same time, however, privacy accepted sexual promiscuity as a satisfactory norm. It forgave it and prevented moral inference by seeing promiscuity as a release (for a long time the only release) of the animal nature we could not avoid in ourselves. Privacy forced us into social patterns and habits of repression that, although founded in the body, affected our intellectual and emotional stature as well for generations to come.

Punishment ritualized pain and dehumanized it. If the body could not truly rid itself of pain, it would, instead, be a party to the glorification of pain. Punishment was to be sought and endured and anticipated because pain could be inflicted, through punishment, as an intellectual challenge to the body. The body would, of course, succumb to its senses, the intellect would win the challenge and therefore claim its dominion over the body. Punishment proved to us that the body was truly worthy of our disdain.

Privacy and punishment, rather than making physicality remote, cornered the body so that it simply became subversive. It had had its loyalties severed, its beauty and health undermined, its place in the person denied it. In attempting to turn our faces away from the physical, towards emotion and mind, we succeeded in emphasizing our bodies and, by the way, our animality. The body became prominant because we wished it not to be there. It became uncontrollable because we tried to tame it.

Science, religion and the literal body

It was widely known and accepted that the body was the site of intellect and emotion, and a belief grew up that to diminish one's physicality would make these 'higher' aspects of our nature more pronounced. So began an era in which social and religious refinements were established to enforce the distance between the physical person and the mental and emotional person.

Cultural experiments in class structure and socio-economic environment were conducted upon the body but without consideration for it. Bodies were counted and categorized. Called 'miserable' when describing the diseased and working bodies of the poor and uneducated. Named 'debauched' — drunken, overfed, lusty — when housing the wealthy and articulate. The body was bedraggled or corsetted, grimy or powdered, yet always debased. Social goals were intellectual in their nature and considered the body very little. Achievement and refinement were described as mental pursuits and purported to 'cleanse' one of one's own physicality. Religion ascribed to a fashionable melancholia, a rather feeble form of emotionalism and was entirely disdainful of physical needs and desires. The body, during this period, was used, abused and abhorred.

This era of refinement ran its course — then bumped to a halt — and the issue that raised its head yet again was pain. Pain from hunger and neglect, pain from lack of shelter and clothing and sanitation, pain from overwork. We didn't seem to have come very far. This pain resembled that of our early ancestors. We thought we had left it behind and moved on to better things so we looked querulously at our work, our environment, our class groupings. We listened more critically to our religious leaders, we reassessed social motives and modes of measurement, then slowly instigated a cultural shift of emphasis.

We knew the body's needs and how to fulfill them, we simply hadn't given enough time to them. Our deep preoccupation with intellect and reason had prevented that. Now we realized that we could not entirely ignore the body, that we must allocate more of our efforts to its care, but, because what we wanted most was to continue our intellectual pursuits, it seemed most prudent to simply give the body what it needed and get on with our thoughts again.

So, we created the 'literal' body: the body without idealized parts or auras or purpose, the body that was simply there to contain us while we observed life and thought our great thoughts. We could take care of this body with the least amount of intellectual involvement. This body could sustain us without interrupting us.

The literal body enabled us to reinforce our class systems, our moral attitudes and our working patterns — all of the so-called achievements of the era of refinement. But, at the same time, the literal body enabled us to open up a new and intellectual endeavour to improve physical health and environment: the scientific endeavour.

Science organized the body. It mechanized it and made it public. Science established a brittle framework of empathy that standardized what was similar between us. It named and attributed all that we were to formulae that were both inflexible and insensitive. Science robbed us of our physical confidence by creating a keeper of the body that was not ourselves. It dictated, in effect, that all sensation,

all movement, all function, must comply with the edicts of science before being truly validated. It was no longer sufficient to sense or feel or function in one's own way and with one's own understanding. Now the body was formal, and it belonged to science.

Science insisted that its literal view of the body would replace all that we despised about the physical world. All animalness, all chaos and all that we could not articulate would now be packaged within the scientific endeavour. It also promised — and achieved — widespread improvements in health.

The precision with which science acted upon the body enabled success in its struggle against disease. Science was entirely intellectual, acting upon the physical, and emotion became invisible to it. No one disputed the presence of soul or emotion within the person, but there was simply no room for its vague features in the formulae that were the foundations of science. With one or two brief exceptions, the mood of science was towards fragmentation of the physical world to enable understanding of it. Understanding of this sort facilitated control, control could guarantee health, health ensured the success and furtherance of society.

Humankind was still raising its head. We had fallen and stumbled and chafed ourselves over thousands of years. We knew we had further to go. Science appeared to help us.

The control that science wielded built a dense framework for our lives so that, more and more, we functioned in a regimented fashion. The mechanization, the literalness, intended for our bodies seeped through to our hearts and minds. We lost our fluency with adaptation, creativity and compassion. We closed ourselves off from other peoples, other points of view, other channels of thought.

The world divided in the same way that we ourselves had divided. As we fragmented our bodies, so we sectioned off the world; as we created formulae for our bodies, so we formalized and structured the life around us. What was started to preserve health became a compulsive, blind urge. But regimentation worked: it pulled us out of pestilence into a relative state of health, physical health.

Healthy, wealthy and lost

Physical health from science has made a tremendous difference to millions of people over many generations and throughout many countries. We can expect a longer life, one less peppered with illness, and we may, if we apply ourselves, expect greater personal accomplishment during our lives. But our most recent history shows humankind suffering from a deeper, more powerful disease than we have ever before confronted.

The wound we inflicted upon our psyche — that of denying true value and relationship between body, mind and emotion — dug too deeply for too long. We were successful, accomplished, dominating, but we had lost our selves. We created a potential for progress — actually invented the concept — but then slipped into a retrogressive spiral of violence and insularity.

True humanity, true empathy left us. The ability to 'value another as you would value yourself' was replaced with 'dog-eat-dog' attitudes that subscribed to the very animality we had worked so hard to avoid. While life and freedom were being espoused by the voices of science and regiment, a filth of violence smudged our healthy hands.

Violence to equality and the desire for community surfaced in world wars and the exploitation of class structures. Violence to the beauty of opposite and balance and creation grew potent through pornography and increased suppression of womanhood and all that implied the feminine. Violence to thought and feeling and even progress itself flourished in our consistent devaluation of ourselves, in our loss of empathy and compassion for others and in our refusal to free ourselves from the regimented, literal, mechanical bondage we had imposed upon our bodies. Violence upon violence in a state of health.

Early generations knew that we are three essences: body, mind and emotion. Later, some cultures came beautifully close to what may be called balance — placing equal importance on these essences and sustaining their relationship. But always, throughout our history, we have been handicapped by some aspect of our immaturity. Something has always happened that prevented the complete, possibly brief, balancing that enables essences to meld into one. We have always, unfortunately, been a flower in bud, not blossom.

We arrive in the present with our inheritance of body, but it is a sorry sight. We are diseased with loss: loss of knowledge and awareness and trust in our bodies; loss of exuberance and joyousness; loss of empathy and communicative abilities; loss of compassion; loss of love.

The body in our lives today
Kidnap, ransom and rescue

You have been kidnapped. It happened in one moment when you were positioned, shaped, clothed or controlled to suit someone else. For you that moment was the first rupture of self-confidence, the first tremor in your understanding of your self and in that moment you were stolen from your potential.

Society's efforts to focus you into productive, useful occupation has robbed you of your own personal motivation. Society's need to establish parametres of behaviour and direction has blinded you to your own unique perspective. Society's compulsion to measure social progress and achievement has inhibited your individual progress and curtailed your unique achievements. Society force-feeds an assumption: You can't do everything.

You believe that and so you gradually stop trying new activities. You do what comes 'naturally' and concentrate on being effective, successful, good at what you do. Being good at something is a very comfortable position to be in but there is sometimes a drawback: when you become more and more accomplished at your successes, you may become more bereft of courage and spontaneity. Your peer group, your colleagues, your style of clothing, your level of stress may begin to curtail your curiosity and your urge to explore. You soon become limited in what you are able to do precisely because you have limited what you are willing to try.

Work and play

You are your own society, your own peer group. You place constraints upon your body to ensure that it conforms to the life-style you have assumed for it. You make a cliché of your body, coerce it to take on the characteristics of an occupation and train it to respond favourably to stimuli with which you are familiar and ignore or refute all stimuli outside your current experience. You find yourself 'kidnapped' from your body and then support that very situation by limiting your actions to suit, which means that your work, your play, your manner of expression all derive from external pressures and impositions that you have, in spite of yourself, agreed to. Look at an example.

Imagine that you have just accepted an administrative or middle management job — anything from Head of Department at a school to Manageress of the Catering Department to Director of Sales. In this sort of work it is important to exude an air of power and control, one of boundless energy for the job with perhaps an element of aggression. Your new role is one of decisiveness, expertise and straight-line thinking. Your clothing must depict these traits and the decor and placement of furniture in your office must create a definite theatre for your effective display of them.

One of the most powerful means of displaying your executive traits is through your own movements and postures. These must be those most likely to reinforce your decisive, expert, cerebral characteristics — both in your own mind and in the minds of your colleagues and subordinates, your 'audience'.

There is nothing new about these movements and poses, however — they are clichés. They are movement patterns that may be quickly transcribed and taken up. Ambitious young bodies, who may have little or nothing in common with the personality these movements depict, or anyone who wishes to become more successful in their particular job arena, may school themselves in a few basic movement techniques.

Try these simple poses and movements and see for yourself:

- Seated: rest your arms wide of body, your feet facing forwards and your back held straight. To show that you are listening, clasp your hands behind your head, displaying your underarm region. If you are female in this role you might, instead, run your fingers slowly through your hair.
- Standing: spread your legs wide apart in a stance. Let your arms hang straight and loose by your sides, or fold them tightly across your chest. From the front, you will look secure and firmly established with no indication of hesitance or discomfort. (In fact, this is an extremely tense pose that is virtually one dimensional in its theatrical effect. That same pose, viewed from the side, is one of precarious imbalance, unsuitable for change, flexibility or progress.)
- Sitting or standing: hold your jaw quite tight (this will probably cause headaches) with nearly clenched teeth. Keep your lips fairly immobile

while talking. Now practice walking — quite heavily with your heels hitting the ground first. When you walk, allow very little movement in your pelvis (this will ultimately cause chronic lower back pain), don't let your arms swing very much and thrust your chin forwards and slightly downwards. As an administrator, you should carry your weight in your shoulders, which will round your upper back. Once this roundness is established, you will need to 'kick' with your shoulders when making a point.

Once these simple variations are learned, you will have little difficulty in dispensing with opinions, emotions, trains of thought and leisure activities that no longer seem in keeping with your new role.

Your 'new' body will see no need for its 'old' details. It will offer no support for them. Support is only offered to those characteristics — whether physical, mental or emotional — that reiterate your new role on all fronts. Your success and longevity in this new occupational role relies heavily on your ability to totally assume the movements and poses of the profession, both in work and play, and at some cost to your previously held emotional, mental and physical styles.

From rubber-band fights in the office right through to the squash courts, the executive mode of play simply re-emphasizes your new use of movement and pose. Now your leisure reinforces aggression, rigidity and no-show emotions. Now your leisure tends to 'play' the part of you that is already most alive: your brain. The result is a steady spiral of depletion in which your physical and emotional repertoire is minimized and made virtually inactive. In your new job, your mind is both worker and player. Intellect and cerebration are all powerful.

You have been kidnapped into a cycle of constraint. Your occupation evolves during your upbringing and gradually shapes your movements and postures. Or, conversely, long-term use of your body in one particular way will identify you into an occupation and when you adhere to one occupation, one mode of life — in work and play — you find yourself constrained, stuck with the same closed view of yourself, the same rigidity, the same reactions from others, the same unchanging body, the same unchanging point of view.

Value, meaning and emotion

The object and purpose of society for the recent millenium has been to spearhead change for the sake of humankind and their continued subsistence on the earth. The last forty years in particular have honed and sharpened this spearhead of progress. We have come to a pinnacle of human application and endeavour, but we have unintentionally burst the bubble of our achievement. We are no longer the same culture we built the rules for.

The process of socialization is based on achievement and limitation. You are taught that achievement results in social acceptance and a sense of personal worth. To achieve, you are taught, you must firstly limit yourself: you must narrow and focus your efforts and your attentions. Then, in order for this achievement-through-limitation to occur, you must prioritize. That is, you must decide precisely which limitations will enable you to attain the greatest achievements. You may then simply live out those limitations in order to achieve your goals.

Over the years, a very clever way of teaching old priorities to new people has developed. It's called convention and it takes the personal out of personal experience and personal values. For example, every country has a convention regarding which side of the road a motorist should drive on. You could choose to drive on the other side, but you would risk collision with another vehicle, resulting in possible injury or death to yourself or others. You and I know this risk. We both accept the list of priorities backing this convention: human life is very important, personal property is important, and so on. However, the experience that created those priorities was someone else's experience. It happened years ago. You and I know this and do not seek to test the convention by having the experience ourselves. Instead, we learn of it and teach it to our children because, in a cultural sense, it saves time and effort.

Another example of convention is politeness. This is a very powerful convention because it crosses cultural boundaries, in theory if not in form. Politeness provides a constant monitor of another's behaviour and facilitates continued contact and communication. Great value is placed on politeness and we are taught to feel outrage or embarrassment if someone is impolite towards us, but that value is also someone else's, a value given years ago. We hold it up as our own because to do otherwise would leave us with little claim to personal worth in that situation — we would feel demeaned. We need this convention to masquerade as a 'personal' value, as part of our 'unique' contribution to social and cultural achievement.

If you adhere to conventional modes of behaviour and systems of prioritizing, then you will achieve according to pre-set, conventional guidelines. Having achieved in this way, you will be socially and culturally valuable and therefore go unnoticed. This summary is, I think, true of many people's existence and is not necessarily worthy of comment, except that it is damaging to many of the individuals concerned.

Constantly living up to others' needs, expectations and requirements erodes your personality. Continually complying with previously established modes of behaviour stifles the creative and explorative nature within you, within all of us. Succumbing to cultural norms and social pressures without question or empirical observation forces us, personally and collectively, into a corner, but you and I and our culture no longer fit that corner.

Purely in terms of your body, this socialization process means that you adopt postural and movement patterns that are inappropriate to you. You strive for a body shape and size that is not necessarily suited to you. You communicate, or attempt to, using physical styles that are inadequate to the levels of communication currently essential within this culture. You draw rigid outlines for your health that exclude many aspects of your personality and you forbid outward, physical behaviour that exposes your uniqueness.

As in your experiences of work and play, you find yourself in another cycle of constraint — you are held to ransom. The value you place on your body determines the meaning that you allocate it, determines the purpose and significance you allow it. That meaning reiterates those same values again — a vicious cycle. You end up reinforcing the system of value-setting that got you where you are in the first place.

The one aspect of your personality that could break the cycle is emotion and emotion is caught up in one of the most diabolical conventions of all: a convention that denies it any value. On any given day, most newspapers will have on their front page a paragraph discounting a point of view because it is 'emotive'. This is a value, but an anti-value. At best, it keeps you tightly within your present orbit of constraint. At worst, this anti-emotion value speeds the depletion of your physical and emotional repertoire.

So your body remains a shell-like thing that houses your mind. You remain used and governed by your mental collaboration with old and brutal value systems. Your body and emotions remain robbed of meaning because the values you have accepted are for your *mind* alone.

'Health' practices

There is just one final step on the way to having a completely modern and used body. When you finally arrive at an occupation or career, once you establish values and physical meaning, once you become truly social, then you inflict the greatest and most insulting wound upon your body: you exclude it from all major considerations.

You become cerebral in emphasis, intellectual in your preference, you profess rationality and logicality. Fewer and fewer of your activities and achievements are channelled through your physical experience. The result is a numbness and a loss of balance and perspective. You lose the ability to compare your mental point of view with your physical point of view, which can make you ill.

Rationality and logic have a small place in wellness. They are by-products of this culture and tools for the promulgation of the mind-over-matter mythology. Your mind, by itself, cannot make your body well. Even mind working together with body cannot make your body well.

Wellness depends on a balance between body, mind *and* emotion within you. Such a balance creates self-trust: a trust in your body, your mind and your emotions. Self-trust is the guardian of your health. It is a constant monitor of wellness and a reliable informant of illness.

Health and illness belong to you, to no one else. Self-trust is yours, balance is yours, but only if your body is yours. And today it isn't so for most people.

We gave up our bodies 200 years ago and we have done very little as a culture to get them back. Modern health is selfless: it is packaged for the millions. It is not *for* you, it is done *to* you — whether it comes out of bottles and boxes or from clinics. It is a practice based on mediocrity and common denominators where your health is 'general' because you are treated just like anyone else. This is so very far from those first feelings of 'having in common' that were the birth of empathy and community in our forebears.

Modern health is irresponsible. It fragments you so that confusion and lack of confidence sit with you in the patient's chair. It places blame onto one fragment of you and gives sentence to another. Modern health allows you to deny involvement with your own health and forces someone else to take up involvement for you. It prefaces its formulae with 'nothing personal' and it means it. Modern health is not for you. Just look at a few modern 'health' practices:

- Fitness: fitness training is based on formulae that categorize you according to age, weight, height, sex, and activity level. But you are never asked if you are a young 39 or an old 24. You are never allowed to add mental or emotional criteria to the formula. You are never, in fitness training, interpreted as a unique individual and helped in establishing your own sense of fitness or wellness. Fitness training is brutal, ritualized pain.

- Dieting: is an extension of, or prelude to, fitness training and involves a significant, sometimes severe, alteration in your eating and nutritional patterns. Sold under the auspices of health, dieting is actually the opposite. It is usually an attempt to help you conform to the current idolization of thinness and can have drastic, sometimes permanent, ill-effects on your metabolism and certain of your major organs.

  Real diet is a way of life. It is a celebration of life through food and eating. It is an approach to wellness that involves other life forms and, as such, ought really to command a profound and respectful relationship between yourself and the food you select.

- Therapy: most therapies tend to select one aspect of your personality and exploit it for the sake of the others. For instance, physical therapies often use the body as a fall-guy in order to reach your mind or emotions. Psychotherapies use your mind to reach — usually — your emotions, and sometimes your body.

  Therapies are generally damaging to some part of you, if only because they are incomplete. They tend to 'rob Peter to pay Paul', an unhealthy practice in any context. The real meaning of therapy is to heal, not to disguise the problem in another form. Healing must result in health or else it's not healing. And there is no health with the imbalance and deceit born out of transporting problems from one part of you to another.

- Drugs: there are more than 25,000 drugs on the market. A very few of them heal, the rest are there to confuse you and your body. Drugs — synthetic, manufactured, branded — add layers of illness to your initial problem. Like therapies, they give a sneaky payoff to one part of you while another part suffers. Drug usage can have a brutal effect on your body. Your symptoms are often shuffled from part of your body to another — for as long as you allow it to continue. With certain drugs, though, your mind and emotions are included in the shuffle, often resulting in depression, nervousness and confusion — to name a few.

When your emotions and intellect become affected by drugs intended for your body, a sort of personality-paralysis occurs that can push you into a false harbour and leave you there. At this point the effects of physical illness, and the illness itself, may become deep and possibly irrevocable.

Your body produces its own drugs and usually in the right proportions. Should the need arise, go to a homoeopathic doctor or a naturopath. These people, if they are well qualified, will look at you as a whole person. They will help you to achieve real balance, which is real health.

● Surgery: some surgery is ritualized pain, for instance, unnecessary episiotomies. Other surgery may be simply a lack of trust in the integrity of the body and a disbelief in its relationship with mind and emotion, both of which have healing powers. A small proportion of the surgery done today is necessary and — in *those* instances *thank goodness for it*.

Surgery is hard on every part of you. Avoid it if you can and, if you can't, then keep in close touch with your homoeopath, who will be able to provide remedial guidance throughout your recovery.

The practices in this list harm your body to various degrees and have very little to offer your mind and emotions. They are advocated as forms of rescue, as a way out when the going gets tough. But, rather than a way out, they are usually a buy out. They all entreat you to give responsibility for your body to someone else: they all encourage and support a mistrust of your self, they are all based on 'spend' rather than 'invest', on 'ignore' rather than 'attend to'.

We are fortunate, today to have means of rescue at all. Science has saved lives, has rescued health, has lengthened our view, even if it hasn't broadened it, and social and cultural history has provided an impressive collection of insights into the trials and errors humankind has endured.

From here, from this moment, your motives and your methods must be those of appropriateness. Many people are working and playing in a fashion that is inappropriate to them. You may be one of them. Many are subscribing to values and adhering to meanings that are often no less than violence to themselves and quite often to those around them. Many are trapped into denying the value and in some cases the presence of emotion, at high cost to all concerned. Many, many people are suffering grave ill-health as a result of cumulative inappropriateness.

This final cycle of constraint robs you of health, then responsibility, then self-awareness.

Appropriateness is a lifeline to balance. It reinstates responsibility and belief in your own ability to grow and establish relationships between yourself and others but, more importantly, within yourself. You are your own society, you are your own, and only, hope of rescue from the backlog of error. You may have come tremendous distances in your life, all the while avoiding balance, but you can go no further. There is a centre, a stillness, within you that needs attention. . .now.

Crucial changes starting now!
The future just happened

By the time you finish reading this sentence, you will be living in the future. Everything you think and feel and do during these split seconds — right now — is your present. And the present is, in fact, your own potential, your own emerging future.

You probably have a tendency to plan, project, anticipate or wait for things to change, events to happen, improvements to occur, but change, like the future, is what you are doing and thinking and feeling right now and again now, and now and now. . .

Change is a natural state. It is your response to a fluctuating world. Change is honest, exciting, rewarding and beneficial. You might feel certain, at times, that it has been inflicted upon you, but actually change is always yours to make appropriate to yourself.

In the next sections and chapters you will begin a process of appropriation. You shall learn how to make change personal to you when you encounter it and you shall learn to initiate change with the aim of improving your physical, mental and emotional selves. You can direct your own progress. You can make change appropriate to you on every level. Right here, right now, is where your present ends. You have just stepped into the future.

Changing your body

You are stuck with it. It's the only one you've got or that you are going to get. It's yours 24 hours a day, every day of your life, whether you like it or not. Do you like it?

You already know how old or young you are, how thin or fat, what shape and size, what ills you've got. There is really no need to talk any further about those particulars unless you want to change them. You may set a fresh starting point for yourself by changing and making a game out of change. You can learn to like yourself and your body very quickly and easily. Here's how.

Game 1

There are three ways in which your body is involved in your life:

- In the way you make use of your body
- By its physical details and characteristics
- In the image or mental picture you hold of it

To start, simply observe yourself over the next 24 hours. Watch how you use your body: how you walk, sit, stand, sleep, work, eat and so on. And notice the details of your body, even if you think they are awful. Just think about them — your feet, your back, your face — focusing on whatever you are doing at the time.

Then notice the image or mental picture you have of yourself. This will vary quite a lot depending on what you are doing. You always hold a mental picture, and you always have some degree of control or influence over its precise nature. By simply taking note of it, you will begin to gain awareness of the importance it plays in your life.

To summarize: for one day just take notice of yourself without being judgmental, without having a tantrum or ending up in the doldrums because you see things you don't like. Just stay calm and look. If it will help, and for some people it can, you might try writing down key words regarding your observations. But whether writing or just thinking your observations, keep clear the distinctions between the three ways in which your body is involved in your life: use, detail and image.

Next day, move on to the second 'change game'.

Game 2

During this 24 hour period all you have to do is decide whether you feel the way you use your body, the details of it, and your image of it are pleasing, displeasing or neither. So, continue in a relaxed fashion with Game 1, but now give each of your observations a 'score': pleasing, displeasing or neither. You may wish to record some of these scores on paper, although it is enough to make a mental note of them.

Just a word here: if you do something more than once in a day, don't observe it once and score it once and then ignore it. Observe it and score it every time you do it. What you see and what you score may well change, that's part of the game.

Game 3

The third game also lasts for 24 hours. Throughout this day, continue with Game 1 and Game 2 — observing and scoring — but automatically pick out every use or detail or image of your body that scores 'displeasing'. Every time one of these comes up, stop doing it right now! Do something else instead.

If you find your use of your body displeasing, then stop using it in that way, *right now*. Is it displeasing to sit in that certain way on your sofa? Then sit on the floor or use cushions to help change your position on the sofa. Is it displeasing to stand talking on the phone the way you always have done? Then lean your back against the wall as you talk.

If you find your self-image displeasing, then refuse to accept that image. Are you displeased with the picture you have of yourself as shy? Then throw out the image. Every time it comes into your head replace it with, for instance, an image of yourself having a good belly laugh. If your self-image depicts you as uncoordinated and you find that displeasing, then stop viewing yourself as uncoordinated. When that image rears its displeasing head, give it a very co-ordinated left then right bat round the ears! Imagine yourself dancing instead.

If you are displeased with the details of your body, then change them if you can. If the fact that you are brunette instead of blonde or fat instead of thin displeases you, then you must replace that displeasure with action: you can dye your hair blonde and you can lose weight. But if your displeasure comes from being only five foot tall. . .well, you know that you can't really alter your height so here you come up against the unchangeable. Even that is a good thing because if you are changing the things you can change and want to change, then those very few things that you cannot change become less displeasing.

If you repeat these three games just once each week for about four weeks, you will experience a gradual but significant increase in positive images of yourself. You will find yourself making good use of your body and you will notice changes in your body details — for instance, loss of excess weight and better posture — which will support good health and a continuing cycle of change and improvement.

Change is a natural state. It is your route to health and maturity. Every change you are able to instigate or be part of, however miniscule it seems, is part of your emerging potential, your future.

Changing your mind

Your mind is an image-maker and a source of volition. These two attributes parent all other manifestations of your mind: opinion, rationality, memory, thought, communication, reason, and so on. For the moment, fix on just these two concepts — image and volition — and you will learn a technique to gain control over your mind's output. This technique is a 'search-and-destroy' mission to pick out negative, obsolete and inappropriate signals from your mind. You may then replace them with positive, relevant and appropriate images, choices and decisions (volition). The aim is, of course, to change. Change to healthy manifestations of mental function. Although this technique is game-like, it is also more tiring than the body-games of the previous section, so use each game for only one hour rather than 24.

Game 1

Look first at the concept of volition: the use of choice and decision. This attribute has been acclaimed as the characteristic that makes us human and separate from other life forms. Yet how much do we know of it? How well do we use it? This mind-game requires that you record, for one hour, all the choices and decisions you make. It doesn't matter what sort of choices they are, or how important the decisions are to you. Choices and decisions are present in quantity during every waking moment of your life. The first step in understanding mental processes is in recognizing them as they are made. So, for just one hour, make note of choices and decisions using the following categories:

- 'Yes' and 'No' decisions: such as 'shall I have lunch with that person?'
- Choices made from multiple options: such as 'shall I sit up and read, go for a late evening walk, ring my brother or have a hot bath and go to bed?'

- Potential for choice and decision created through force of will: such as 'I am unhappy here but I'm going to continue this work until I finish my evening courses, then I'll start out on my own.'

Have a break then try the second mind-game.

Game 2

This game will deal with image. An image is a mental picture, an impression or an idea. It may be contained solely within yourself, in which case it becomes a mental derivative or it may be expressed and communicated — making it a device of the mind. Over the next hour, make note of the images you use and encounter in yourself. Record them in two categories:

- A mental representation that you contain (derivative): such as, the face of a friend appearing in your mind's eye while you are studying.
- A mental representation that you translate (device): such as, you have an idea for a new design that you quickly sketch out for your colleagues to comment upon.

Get used to noticing the manifestations of your mind in this way for four or five days by practising Game 1 and Game 2 once or twice each day. Then add the third mind-game.

Game 3

In this game, watch how your choices and decisions can determine the images you sustain and, vice versa, how the images you sustain determine the choices and decisions you make.

During one hour send a message to yourself — a mental picture — saying that you are ugly, horrible, boring and wicked. At the same time, watch closely the choices you make during that hour and make note of them. You won't enjoy this hour, but it will be revealing.

Rather than taking a break, move straight on to the reverse of this by creating a mental picture of yourself as beautiful, wonderful, interesting and good. Send this message to yourself for one hour also, although it will feel so good you may want to do it for longer. Again, watch closely the choices and decisions you make during this time and make a note of them.

These images are either positive or negative messages. And their effects on your volition (choice and decision) are either positive or negative. Once you have experienced this powerful relationship between image and volition, you may begin to use it. By modifying your mental images, and then exercising volition based on those new images, you may infuse positiveness into your mind — and your life.

When you are first trying these games, you will probably use contained imagery — images that are mental derivatives and therefore stay in your head. However, you may, after a time, wish to use images that you translate or communicate. Images of this sort are mental devices, quite literally tools for your work, your hobbies, your relationships. If you are able to create positiveness in these images, you will begin to create tangible, practical and significant changes in the course your life takes, changes that you have chosen and decided upon.

Explore the effects of positive and negative imagery on each of the three key manifestations of volition listed in the first of these mind-games: yes and no, multiple choice, force of will. You will gradually gain understanding of these mental processes and that understanding will allow you to incur changes in your life that are appropriate to you.

Changing yourself for the better

'Better' is a judgmental and qualitative term, but that is allright. You have a right to your feelings; you are an emotional creature.

If you were to try and convince yourself that you are not emotional, that emotions are unimportant in your life or that you could ever get by without them, then you would be committing a great deceit. As you may recall from previous discussion, deceit creates illness. Emotion is as essential to your well-being as is air or food or sleep or companionship. You must allow emotion in yourself if you wish to attain a healthy and balanced state. And the best and easiest way to allow emotion is to first observe it in yourself. Here's how:

Game 1

Pick an emotion, a really obvious one like anger. Now find another emotion, a more subtle one such as calm. (You should pick emotions that are fairly relevant to you today.) Think about both emotions for a whole day. Just observe how they move in and out of your life during that 24 hour period and get to know as much as you can about them. Keep a record of the day if you like. Include in your record observations about how clearly you think or how your stomach feels while you're angry, or in love, or sad. Don't use your head, just react and be emotional.

Game 2

The following day, choose a different obvious emotion and a different subtle emotion. Watch both of those for the next 24 hour period and, again, make a record of what you observe. You may repeat this process two or three times more, as long as you feel the emotions you are watching are active in yourself. Try not to pretend — if an emotion isn't with you on that particular day, then observe another or have a break. Gradually you will become highly tuned to the presence and strength of emotion in yourself and, by the way, in others.

To allow emotion you must simply acknowledge it and become familiar with how it pertains to your life. Allowing emotion does three things:

- It puts negative and positive emotions in balance.
- It relieves the discomfort of holding back or holding in emotion.
- It enables you to change — change your body, change your mind and change yourself for the better.

Emotion is good. It is crucial to real health and enables your body and mind to function at their optimum levels. Emotion is with you already, it interacts with your mind and body. You do not need to engage in emotional therapy or self-assessment or catharsis to rediscover it for yourself. But be aware: there are many myths and taboos concerning emotion. If you subscribe to them, these myths can hold you back and prevent you from reaching your potential. Most noticeable is the taboo that encourages you to hide your emotion under the auspices of mind.

You have, by now, undoubtedly developed an ability to observe yourself: your body, your mind and your emotions. You have probably learned quite a lot, too, about how your body, mind and emotion functions. I hope you have set yourself a few goals, a few changes you would like to make to each of these aspects of your personality.

Using your observations, your goals and the movement designs that follow, you can strengthen the relationships between your body, your mind and your emotions. You can initiate the changes that are essential to health, maturity, and attainment of personal potential.

Start now, because your future has just happened.

Chapter 3

Gaining insight — your body speaks

Have you ever been to one of those meetings where one or two people monopolize the discussion? Everyone else sits there feeling cross, cynical or bored. Some people may even get up and leave — thinking either that they aren't necessary to the success of the meeting or that they would do well to avoid such unpleasant and haphazard occasions in future. But decisions are made and things do happen as a result of such assemblies. The reason is, usually, that those same one or two people bulldoze their way forward until they get what they want.

Imagine yourself observing the meetings described below. In each meeting, there are only three people and, though they don't know it, each person is as important as the other two in determining the meeting's outcome.

Meeting 1: in the alley

This meeting takes place in an alley to decide how to divide some money between three men. Mr. M begins to speak but Mr B hits him in the mouth, so Mr M keeps quiet. Mr E begins to cry because now he is frightened. Mr B doesn't like crying so he hits Mr E in the mouth, too. Mr M and Mr E look at one another and allow Mr B to divide the money anyway he wants to.

Meeting 2: in the boardroom

This meeting is being conducted in a very plush boardroom to decide whether to spend some money on a new project. Mr M is doing all the talking, using big words and taking very few pauses for breath. Mr B has some 'morning after' symptoms and is desperate to go to the toilet, but every time he starts to excuse himself, Mr M tells him to stay until he has finished speaking. Mr E is sitting quietly but feels sorry for Mr B so Mr E tries to interrupt Mr M's flow of words but he, too, gets silenced. Mr B and Mr E look at each other and quickly agree with Mr M's proposals so that they may end the meeting.

Meeting 3: in the corridor

This meeting takes place by chance in a corridor. Mr M and Mr B are walking together towards a lecture theatre where they are soon to deliver a very important paper. Mr E approaches them. He has a red face, puffy, watery eyes and a slow gait. He holds out his hand and asks the two men, in a sullen voice, if they will give him some money. Mr M and Mr B are preoccupied and so shake their heads. Mr E then begins to shout and swear at them. There are many important colleagues passing Mr M and Mr B. They feel acutely embarrassed by Mr E's outburst and so they give him some money. Mr E stops shouting and swearing and Mr M and Mr B move on.

These are three examples of successful meetings. In Meeting 1, Mr B got his own way and the purpose of the meeting — that the money be divided — was achieved. In Meeting 2, Mr M got his own way and the decision was made about whether or not to go ahead with the funding for a new project. In Meeting 3, Mr E got his own way and the meeting was successful in its conclusion — Mr E was satisfied and went away quietly.

You have probably played each of these three roles yourself at various times and you almost certainly know people who fit the character of each role described above. Now read through the examples again, but this time for Mr B, read Body, for Mr M, read Mind and for Mr E, read Emotion.

In Meeting 1, Body bullies Mind and Emotion. In Meeting 2, Mind ignores Body and Emotion. In Meeting 3, Emotion intimidates Body and Mind. During every waking moment of your life meetings similar to these are being conducted within you. The type of meetings, their frequency and your management of them denote your personality. Your personality is a meeting of Body, Mind and Emotion.

If you could draw personality, if you could draw this meeting, it might appear as three persons seated around a triangular table: each person and their side of the table representing body, mind or emotion. But how many ways are there of drawing a triangle? How great is the variety of personalities? Look at these triangular representations of the meetings sited earlier.

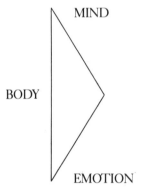

Meeting 1: Emphasis is Body

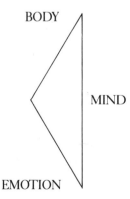

Meeting 2: Emphasis is Mind

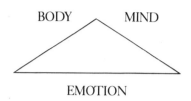

Meeting 3: Emphasis is Emotion

These drawings depict imbalance. In each of them, one of the triangle's sides is longer than the other two sides. In each, one aspect of the personality is made dominant because it, literally, takes up more space. But there is another way of looking at these meetings.

Imagine that the drawings above are single frames in a strip of film. If you show them, one after the other, at high speed, the three triangles will blur together to appear as one triangle with equal sides. Slow the film down again and you can observe the dominant side shifting from Body to Mind to Emotion and then round again.

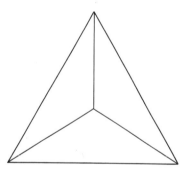

Let's think of this in terms of another meeting:

Meeting 4: at the auction rooms

This is a pre-arranged meeting to invest money for some important clients of B, M & E. Mr M arrives at the auction rooms first and begins to work on the days valuations. Mr E arrives next and comes to Mr M to receive verbal instructions. Mr M goes into these at length, by which time Mr B has arrived and positioned himself at his vantage point on the floor.

The auction is announced and, when items included in his instructions come up, Mr E signals to Mr B who begins to bid. Acting on the instructions signalled to him, Mr B is able to purchase several items for investment. As the morning progresses, Mr E moves swiftly around the auction rooms, he notes the purchases made and informs Mr M, who is keeping track of the company's expenditure. Mr E listens to Mr M's new instructions, then signals these to Mr B who, by this time, is bidding on another item. At lunch, Mr B, Mr M and Mr E sit together over a delicious meal to celebrate a good morning's work and the success of their collaboration.

In Meeting 4, B, M & E got its own way, Mr B, Mr M and Mr E got their own way and the important clients got their own way. Meeting 4 was the most successful of the meetings because every person, at every stage of the exchange, achieved their goal.

Now look at the triangular representation for Meeting 4.

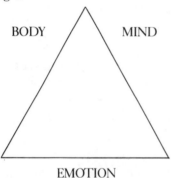

In this triangle, emphasis is shared between Body, Mind and Emotion because, in the meeting, there was collaboration between these three elements. The result? All sides become equal. As in the film strip, if you had stopped Meeting 4 before its conclusion, you could have drawn one of the first three triangles — at one moment emphasizing Mr B, the next Mr M, the next moment Mr E — but it is the results or the culmination of this meeting that we must consider now. Meeting 4 was the most successful for all concerned. This was achieved, firstly, through equal and obvious importance being given to each of the three characters. And secondly, by each character, each side of the triangle, performing only those actions that were appropriate to its own capabilities.

Surely what you hope and imagine for yourself is an internal Meeting 4: a personality that is balanced, active and effective. A personality that is unified in its aims and achievements. An equilateral triangle. Yet how is this possible?

Look at this final drawing of a disjointed triangle.

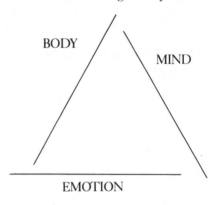

If you take each side of this triangle, each aspect of your personality, and look closely at it alone, you may discover which of your activities and endeavours are appropriate to it. You may gain a greater understanding of your personality as it functions. You may establish an internal Meeting 4 for yourself.

Your body the actor

All that you think, hope for, imagine or feel is only ever possible, every environment or situation or place is only ever accessible to you because you have a body.

Your body is your form. It must house you and move you and shape you and define you in a physical world. Your body is the outward sign of your life. A visible and vital manifestation of your attributes and your characteristics.

Your body is your experience made tangible. Through it you sense and give expression to all manner of things. It is your means of extending into the world around you. And your body, alone of your three natures, is loose in the world. It is mobile and sentient and outwardly expressive. Your mind and your emotions are united into your body — they are embodied — leaving your body with one definite task.

Your body is an actor. It performs and mimics and simulates, as best it can, the events of mind and emotion. It animates thoughts and feelings. It exerts physical influence to fulfil the needs of mind, emotion and, of course, itself.

Your body has an exhuberance for life: it wants to be an exquisite house for you, a powerful and unique sensor, a great mover — especially to give passionate, precise expression to you. Your body doesn't even care who you are, it does not discriminate, it commits itself to you entirely, it is your best friend and your best friend for life.

Your mind the inhibitor

Does that description surprise you? Perhaps you thought your mind was the least inhibited aspect of your personality -- not necessarily so.

Inhibition is an integrant function of mind, though it undertakes this duty in the most comforting way it knows. Your mind welcomes any and all information and stimuli. It is greedy and eclectic, but it says, 'wait in line, queue up in this order, tell me what you are and I will remember you, make your statement as clear and distinct as possible, don't go — all of you will be given my attention.' Your mind inhibits the natural qualities of the stimuli it receives in order to focus and control those qualities; it is a processing plant through which all of the information it receives must pass before being given over to body or emotion.

The mental process is a powerful set of rules. And your mind is obsessed with implementing them — tirelessly, repeatedly, compulsively. The rules are simple: gather, prioritize, memorize, synthesize. And, of course, your mind complies with its own rules extremely well! It loves to collect information. It naturally establishes that information in an order of importance. It plays with recall and delights in making information accessible to you. Left to itself, your mind would probably not rate either your body or your emotions very highly: they are too full of surprises, too inconsistent in their characters. And so, not surprisingly, your mind tends to place itself first on its list of priorities.

The rules and inhibitions wrought by your mind usually work to your advantage, to the benefit of your body and emotions as well as your mind. Because your mind finds patterns in all information and shows them to you. It throws images and likenesses up from its memory. It creates avenues of approach for your ease in assimilating the information it has gathered and it defines that information for you over and over again. It never becomes impatient, it never turns from a challenge. Your mind is positive and, by its own laws, certain.

Emotion the communicator

Everything you experience is felt by your emotions. Nothing that happens to you, nothing that you do or think, goes without notice from them and very little of it occurs at all without their involvement.

Emotion completes an invisible circulation between body and mind. It is always between them and is essential to them both. The work of translation, relation, and communication are its commitments and it attempts to perform these in the nature of an emollient: softly.

Emotion understands two languages apart from its own: the body's and the mind's. It understands them both entirely, without prejudice or favour and it is therefore a constant endeavour of emotion to translate each of these languages into the other. Whatever signals are sent between body and mind are first translated by emotion so that body and mind may respond to one another and this response is translated also.

But there is more: emotion mediates. It says, 'listen to what the other has said. Respond or react, but you can't do without me and I won't let you do anything except get along with each other. I will show you how.' So emotion creates relationship, internal relationship, between body, mind and itself.

As well as understanding three languages, emotion has an excellent comprehension of motivation — that which causes these languages in the first place. There are only two types of motivation: inner and outer. They are both complex in themselves but work together very simply — by another system of prioritization. Emotion governs that system, it barters.

Emotion says, 'listen body, mind has a great need to receive stimulation. What is your greatest need at the moment?' and if body says, 'I'm alright, quite happy', then emotion sets the mind's need as a priority and you get to do something mentally stimulating. If body says, 'no way, I'm tired and hungry', then emotion tells mind to 'wait' while you eat something and take a nap.

If both mind and body are being obstreperous and not budging from their own preferences, emotion still holds the final cards. It says, 'now you've done it. I'm going to override both of your so-called urgent needs.' In this case you may become melancholy and suffer inaction.

Emotion communicates: it imparts sensation, emphasis, need and motivation from one aspect of your personality to another; it repeats itself as often as is necessary to get the message through; it repeats itself even when mind or body don't want to listen; it is the part of you that really wants exchange, that really wants to reach out and to hold close; it is unconditional in its guardianship over you. Emotion is the side of the table, the aspect of your personality, that seeks balance, self-awareness and unity. Emotion is your gift from God.

The measure of yourself

How well do you know your body, your mind, your emotions? Which of the triangular drawings of a few pages back best represents the 'shape' of your personality? Which of the meetings described is most similar to your own behaviour within yourself? What is your own blend of body, mind and emotion? Your body can tell you these things.

There are 12 simple movements described and illustrated over the next few pages. Each of these movements is capable of giving you insight into the relationships at work within you. Each movement will help you to know what proportions of body, mind and emotion comprise your personality. Each will continue the process of change and appropriation begun in Chapter 2. Each movement will make you feel more alive, more alert and more attractive.

Three questions follow the instructions for each movement. One question for body, one for mind and one for emotion. After you have completed the first movement, please answer the Body question that follows. Then complete the second movement and answer the Body question that follows that movement.

Continue in this way until you have completed all 12 movements and answered all the Body questions.

Then go back to the first movement and repeat it, but this time answer the Mind question. Perform all 12 movements again, answering all of the Mind questions.

Finally, repeat the movements a third time but this time answer the Emotion questions. By the time you have repeated the movements three times, you will be quite competent and familiar with them.

To help you recall your response to each question, record your answers on a separate sheet of paper.

MOVEMENT	BODY	MIND	EMOTION
One	a	b	c
Two	a	c	c
Three	a	a	b
Four	b	c	a
Five	a	c	b
Six	a	a	c
Seven	c	c	a
Eight	a	c	b
Nine	c	c	c
Ten	b	a	b
Eleven	a	a	b
Twelve	b	c	c

Many of the movements may be performed seated or standing, so if you are handicapped or for some reason confined to a chair or bed, you may still enjoy many of them. You may perform the movements fast or slow, large or small — that is entirely up to you. It is important to perform the movements at least twice. So when an instruction asks you to 'repeat the movement' please perform it once again. If the movement is predominant in its use of one side of your body, when you repeat it please reverse it also. It is possible, in these cases, that you will wish to

perform the movement *twice* on each side of the body. Please feel free to do so — it will only improve your practice and your sense of ease.

Wear what you like so long as you can move in it . . . and enjoy yourself. Remember, you are not exercising, you are not trying to 'get fit', you are moving to gain insight into the meeting of body, mind and emotion that is going on right now within you. You are moving to give voice to each side of the triangle, each aspect of your personality.

The basic 12 movements

MOVEMENT 1:

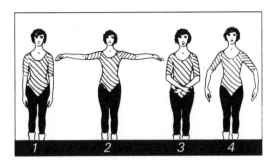

1 Stand in a relaxed manner, or sit upright on the edge of a chair or stool. Keep your shoulders level and your arms hanging straight by your sides.

2 Raise both arms to shoulder level and at the same time take a breath in. Keep your body upright, your neck muscles relaxed, chin and shoulders level and hands relaxed. The palms of your hands should face down.

3 Allow both arms to swing down from their raised position so that they cross in front of you. Do this as you breathe out. Notice which arm crosses in front and which behind the other (reverse this position the next time you perform the movement).

4 Uncross your arms and open them out to either side making a soft, rounded shape with them. Your palms will face in toward your hips and slightly upward. Breathe in as you make this part of the movement. To finish, breathe out and move into position **1**. Repeat the movement.

MOVEMENT 2:

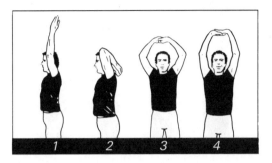

1 Stand tall or sit upright and stretch both arms up over your head. Turn the palms of your hands to face behind you and keep your elbows straight. Hold this position for just a few seconds while you make certain that your chin is level, your neck quite relaxed and that you are breathing!

2 Now fold your arms at the elbows so that your palms face in toward your back. Try and keep your chin level and your neck relaxed. It is important to hold your elbows high, straight up if you can manage. Remember to breathe. You may repeat these two movements if you like.

3 Hook your fingers together up over your head. Now imagine someone is pulling your locked hands up and, at the same time, someone else is pulling your elbows out. This creates a very strong sensation. Breathe.

4 Now stretch your arms straight up over your head again, this time cupping your hands together with both palms upwards. Breathe in as you stretch strongly up, breathe out as you relax the stretch slightly. Repeat.

THE QUESTIONS

BODY: Are you most aware of your:
a) arms b) shoulders c) torso?
MIND: Do you prefer: a) either b) left
c) right arm to cross in front?
EMOTION: Which movement is most relaxing
to you: a) 2 b) 3 c) 4?

THE QUESTIONS

BODY: Are you most conscious of your:
a) muscles b) joints c) breathing?
MIND: Do you see these as a) angular b) round
c) linear movements?
EMOTION: Which hand position do you prefer
a) 1 and 2 b) 3 c) 4?

The basic 12 movements

MOVEMENT 3:

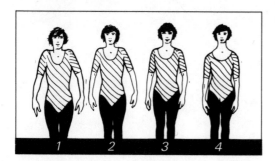

MOVEMENT 4:

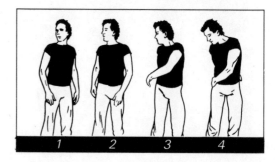

1 Stand or sit and let your arms hang at your sides. Although your arms will move, think mostly of your shoulders and do not let your arms become tense. Now lift your shoulders as far as you can up towards your ears. Breathe in as you do this.

2 Now breathe out in a rather shallow manner as you begin to lower your shoulders. They will be slightly lifted but not shrugged.

3 Still breathing out in shallow puffs, continue to lower your shoulders. They will be just about level in this part of the movement.

4 Still breathing out, in fact, squeezing the last bit of breath out, stretch your shoulders down below the level position. Return to the first position and repeat.

Note: this entire movement may be done slowly and deliberately or in a rapid, punchy manner, which will probably cause you to laugh! In addition, you may add more gradations of the downward movement to those illustrated here. In that case, be certain to give a slight breath out at each point.

1 Stand tall with your feet shoulder-width apart or sit tall on a chair without arms. Keep your shoulders level, your neck and arm muscles relaxed. Now turn your chin to one shoulder.

2 Twist your shoulders and chest in the same direction, allowing your chin to stay put (now it will line up with your sternum). Keep as relaxed as you can, keep breathing, and keep your back straight.

3 Maintain the twist in your upper torso, but now drop your head, shoulders and upper back into a curve. At the same time stretch your arms in front and across your body to deepen both the curve and the twist.

4 Stretch your arms in a continued arc until you are able to place one hand on the back of each hip. So, for instance, if you have curved to the right, your left hand will be gripping your right hip, your right hand will be pressed against the back of your left hip. Hold this position for at least one good breath in and out. Uncurl and repeat on the other side.

THE QUESTIONS

BODY: Are you most aware of your:
a) shoulders b) neck c) arms?
MIND: Which movements are opposites
a) 1 and 4 b) 1 and 3 c) 2 and 4?
EMOTION: Does this movement make you
a) relax b) giggle c) sigh?

THE QUESTIONS

BODY: Do you feel this twist mostly in the region of your: a) pelvis and hips b) ribs and waist c) neck and shoulders?
MIND: In part 4, do you look towards a) one hip b) the floor c) your back?
EMOTION: In part 4, are you most aware of a) breath b) stillness c) twist?

The basic 12 movements

MOVEMENT 5:

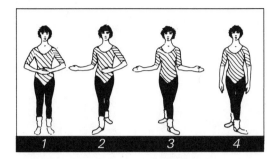

MOVEMENT 6:

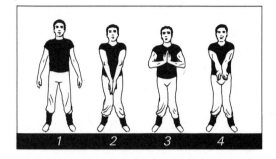

1 Stand with your feet hip-width apart, your toes facing forwards. Now place your fingers over your navel and relax your shoulders. Try to keep your neck and shoulders relaxed and your chin level during all of this move.

2 Take one step forwards and, as you do so, turn that set of toes out to the side. At the same time, 'open' the forearm on that side of your body as if it were a door. Keep your elbow close to your waist. Your palm will now face to the front. Try to keep your hand in a straight line with your forearm.

3 Repeat this on the other side of your body: take a step forward with the toes facing out. At the same time, 'open' the other arm.

4 Now take a smaller step with the first leg so that you stop with your heels close together and both sets of toes facing out. Allow your arms to fall straight, a little distance from your sides. When you are ready, turn your toes forward again and repeat this sequence.

1 Stand tall, or sit, with your feet shoulder-width apart, toes forwards. Hold your arms straight and slightly lifted from your sides. Look forwards with your chin level.

2 Now turn your toes and knees inwards, bending your knees to touch each other. At the same time, wrap your shoulders forwards so that your arms swing together. The backs of your hands should touch. Keep your chin level and breathe.

3 Maintaining the position of your lower body, begin to bring your hands in towards your navel. Keep some pressure between the backs of your hands as you rotate them inwards and upwards, as though turning your arms inside-out.

4 With the same lower-body position, press your forearms and elbows together as you pull out of the rotation. Press the outside edges of your hands together as you complete the rotation. Your palms should turn slightly out, towards your shoulders, like pages of a book. Look into your hands. Keep as much height in your torso as you can manage and breathe.

THE QUESTIONS

BODY: Do you feel this most in your
a) hips b) arms c) feet and ankles?
MIND: What do you find is working hardest, your a) balance b) co-ordination c) attention to detail?
EMOTION: Do you feel a) OK b) silly c) uncomfortable in this move?

THE QUESTIONS

BODY: Are you most aware of your:
a) knees b) hips c) arms and hands?
MIND: Which best describes the movement to you: a) being squeezed from behind
b) being sucked inwards c) being squashed from both sides?
EMOTION: Which part of the movement do you prefer a) 2 b) 3 c) 4?

MOVEMENT 7:   **MOVEMENT 8:**

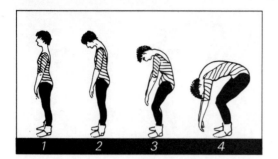

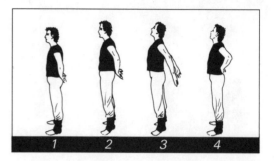

1 Stand or sit with your back straight. Place your feet hip-width apart. Relax your shoulders, arms, neck and level your chin.

2 Drop your chin forwards and pause briefly to feel its weight. As though this weight took control, slowly curl your neck and upper back forwards. Your shoulders and arms will begin to hang forwards of your body.

3 Bend your knees slightly as you continue this forward curl. The head is loose, the neck and arms very relaxed and heavy. Curl forwards until your hands are approximately knee level. In this position your pelvis is still upright. Pause briefly to feel the full weight of your upper body.

4 Now tilt your pelvis forwards so that you complete this curl. Your hands may brush against the floor and your knees will bend more deeply. Hold this position for three or four breaths with complete relaxation in your neck and shoulders. Uncurl from this by reversing the order of positions.

1 Stand or sit tall with your feet hip-width apart and your hands clasped behind at your tail-bone. Keep your chin level, your neck and shoulders relaxed.

2 If you are standing, lift onto tip-toe keeping your ankles straight. At the same time (either standing or sitting), raise your clasped hands behind you to help your balance. You will feel your shoulder blades come together. Maintain the relaxation in your neck and keep your chin level. Breathe.

3 Hold the balanced position while you turn your face towards the ceiling. Expand your chest slightly as you do this and lift your arms higher behind you if you need to. Think of the top of your sternum as another eye 'looking' towards the ceiling.

4 Slowly lower onto your heels again, but keep your chin lifted and your chest open. As you lower your heels, slide your fingers onto the back of your waist. Your elbows will move out to the side, your sternum will remain lifted.

THE QUESTIONS

BODY: Which position gives you the most comfort a) 2   b) 3   c) 4?
MIND: Are you most aware of your spine while a) curling down   b) standing after you have curled down and up   c) curling up?
EMOTION: Would you rather this movement a) went further than position 4   b) ended in position 2   c) ended in position 3?

THE QUESTIONS

BODY: What do you find most challenging about this movement a) balance   b) neck and head position   c) arm position?
MIND: In positions 2, 3 and 4, are you most aware of your a) hands   b) chin   c) chest?
EMOTION: Which best describes position 4 for you a) awkward   b) proud   c) vulnerable?

The basic 12 movements

MOVEMENT 9:

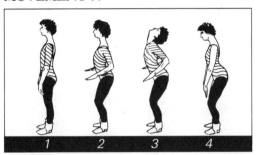

1 Stand or sit tall with your feet hip-width apart. If you are sitting, concentrate on the upper-body element of this movement. Level your chin and relax your arms a little distance from your sides.

2 Reach your tail-bone back to create an arch in the lower back. At the same time, begin to pull your elbows sharply back to create an arch in your upper back. Bend your knees slightly as you arch. Look forwards.

3 Bend your knees as deeply as possible while keeping your heels flat. At the same time, pull your tail-bone and your elbows as far back as possible and turn your face to the ceiling. Keep your elbows about shoulder-height.

4 Maintain the position of your lower back and knees. Now stretch your arms in the direction of your knees. Turn your face to look at your hands.

MOVEMENT 10:

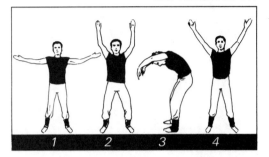

1 Stand with your feet shoulder-width apart and your toes turned slightly out to the side. If you are sitting, concentrate on the upper-body element of this movement. Spread your arms wide at shoulder level with your palms facing forwards and slightly up.

2 Draw your arms up and forwards in a soft, round arc. At the same time, begin to bend your knees and round your lower back. Look forwards.

3 Continue the arc movement of your arms until you have circled them round in front of you, palms facing you, elbows high. At the same time, deepen the bend of your knees and the curve of your entire back. Look towards your knees. Pause here and imagine you are holding a giant ball.

4 Make a sudden, strong movement that stretches your legs, back and arms into an upright, open position. Your arms and legs are shoulder-width apart. Look forwards. Imagine you have just thrown the ball away.

THE QUESTIONS

BODY: What part of your back feels this movement the most: a) lower back and pelvis   b) back of the waist   c) between the shoulders?
MIND: Are you most aware of the a) curve of your back   b) angle of your knees   c) position of your arms?
EMOTION: Do you feel a) silly   b) strong   c) stretched in this movement?

THE QUESTIONS

BODY: Which part of your body works hardest in this complete movement: a) spine   b) shoulders   c) knees?
MIND: Which parts please you most a) 2 and 3   b) 3 and 4   c) 1 and 4?
EMOTION: Do you prefer a) making the ball   b) holding the ball   c) throwing the ball away?

MOVEMENT 11:

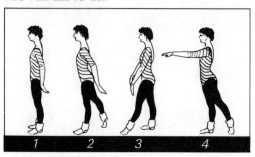

1 Stand with your feet hip-width apart and your arms reaching gently behind you, palms facing back. (If you are in a wheelchair, you may enjoy part of this movement by positioning your chair in a doorway with the jamb slightly behind you. Hold onto the jamb so that your palms face back.)

2 Reach one leg back and step lightly onto your toes. Raise your arms up behind you at the same time. (In a chair, push yourself forward slightly so that your arms are stretched up behind you.)

3 Lower your weight onto your rear leg and draw your arms to your sides, palms backwards. (Pull your chair backwards until you are in the doorway and your hands are in line with your shoulders.)

4 Continue to move backwards: this time take a step with your other leg as you swing both arms forward, palms facing down. (In a chair, continue pushing yourself backwards through the doorway until your arms are in front of you.) Now reverse the entire movement so that you move forwards.

MOVEMENT 12:

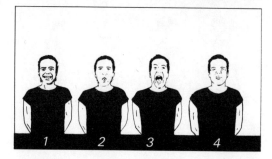

1 Make yourself comfortable. Now spread your mouth sideways to 'bare' your teeth. Aim to shape your mouth into a rectangle.

2 Pull your mouth forwards, the lips forming on 'o', as far as you can. Keep your neck relaxed, it's just your face doing the moving this time.

3 Open your jaw as far as you can and pull your lips back from your teeth. Keep your lower jaw in line with the upper: no side-to-side movements.

4 Pull your chin up, your lips forwards and up towards your nose, your eyes down and together. Aim to put all of your features into as small an area as you possibly can. Repeat these four movements.

Note: Try these without a mirror first — otherwise your may find yourself in a fit of giggles. On the other hand, if you feel in need of hysterical laughter, practice these with your best friend.

THE QUESTIONS

BODY: Are you most aware of your:
a) arm movement b) stepping c) hands?
MIND: Do you think most about your a) balance b) speed c) direction?
EMOTION: Do you a) dislike b) like c) don't mind moving backwards?

THE QUESTIONS

BODY: Which makes the area around your eyes most relaxed a) 1 b) 3 c) 4?
MIND: Which of these would you rather *not* do a) 2 b) 3 c) 4?
EMOTION: Which of these seems funniest to you a) 1 b) 2 c) 4?

When you have performed these 12 movements three times and answered all 36 questions, you may refer to your answer sheet again. Following these guidelines, please put a number beside each of your answers:

BODY questions answered a), give value of 1.
     answered b), give value of 2.
     answered c), give value of 3.
MIND questions answered a), give value of 2.
     answered b), give value of 3.
     answered c), give value of 1.
EMOTION questions answered a), give value of 3.
     answered b), give value of 1.
     answered c), give value of 2.

Here is a sample answer sheet filled in:

MOVEMENT	BODY	MIND	EMOTION	TOTAL
1	a = 1	b = 3	c = 2	6
2	a = 1	c = 1	c = 2	4
3	a = 1	a = 2	b = 1	4
4	b = 2	c = 1	a = 3	6
5	a = 1	c = 1	b = 1	3
6	a = 1	a = 2	c = 2	5
7	c = 3	c = 1	a = 3	7
8	a = 1	c = 1	b = 1	3
9	c = 3	c = 1	c = 2	6
10	b = 2	a = 2	b = 1	5
11	a = 1	a = 2	b = 1	4
12	b = 2	c = 1	c = 2	5
TOTAL:	19	18	21	

You total these values in two ways. First, add up the values vertically so that you arrive at one sum under the BODY column, one under the MIND column, and one under the EMOTION column. (Each of these three totals will be no less than 12, no greater than 36.)

Secondly, total the values across the page so that you arrive at 12 sums — one for each movement. (Each of these 12 totals will be no less than three, no greater than nine). Circle any of these sums that are an eight or nine total.

Now you may use all of these totals to arrive at a three-letter code that will help you to schedule the best Movement Design practice for yourself.

Look again at the totals at the bottom of the page. Find the *smallest* total of the three. Which column is it under? If, for example, it is under MIND then 'M' is the first letter of your code.

What is the next smallest total? If it is the number under the BODY column, then the second letter of your code is 'B'.

What is the *largest* total and which column is it under? In this example, it is under EMOTION. Therefore, the third and final letter of the code is 'E'.

The code is MBE.

Remember, the smallest total gives the first letter, the largest total gives the last letter in your code. You will end up with one of these codes.

BME	BEM	MBE
MEB	EBM	EMB

There is a slight chance that two or even all three totals will be equal. In that case simply put an equals sign between those totals that are equal, for instance: BM = E, MB = E, EB = M, B = ME, M = BE, E = BM or whatever combination is appropriate. The lowest total is still represented in the first letter(s), the highest total in the last letter(s). If your code is one with an '=' between two letters, then you should read two of the summaries below. For instance, if your code is B = ME, then you should read the summary for code BME and code MBE, simply reversing the position of the two equal letters. You must decide which summary most resembles your knowledge of yourself. Then, either follow its guidelines or extend your practice by combining the two summaries and performing the suggested movements for both codes.

In addition, if the '=' is present in your code, you should emphasize those movements from The basic 12 where your total scores equalled eight or nine.

(You should have already circled them, they are the totals on the side of your score sheet.) So, whenever you perform The basic 12 movements, perform them *all* and then repeat those whose totals are eight or nine. Whenever you perform movements from The top 20 in Chapter 5, add The basic 12 movements with an eight or nine score to your practice, too.

Your code will help you to customize your practice of Movement Design, but it is a flexible option. You may wish to alter, extend or curtail your practice according to your own interpretation of your physical, mental and emotional needs at any one time.

Here are the suggested guidelines for each code:

BME   You have a good awareness of your body. Perhaps you are an athletic person or one who enjoys sports, dance or fitness classes. You usually consider your body's needs first in most situations so, in your movement practice you will need to give slightly more attention to the mental and emotional elements of your movements. This shouldn't be difficult for you, because your movements will become more pleasureable as a result.

● Perform all The basic 12 movements once each week throughout your practice.
● Become familiar with The top 20 movements by making the Voyages described in Chapter 5. Take one or two weeks for this.
● Perform movements 2, 6, 12, 15, 16, 17 and 18 from The top 20 twice each week for the next month of your practice. Perform all of The top 20 movements once each week during this time.
● Use the Posy for each movement during two of your top 20 practices; use the Image during the one remaining top 20 practice.

BEM   You also have a strong awareness of your body but you probably use it in an intuitive manner. So, for instance, you may sense the symptoms of a cold or the flu well before they appear, or you may feel 'atmosphere' through your stomach. In your practice you will need to give much of your attention to the mental and emotional elements of your movements, with special focus on the development and control of mental images (see Chapter 2).

● Perform all The basic 12 movements once each week throughout your practice.
● Become familiar with The top 20 movements by making the Voyages drescribed in Chapter 5. Take

one or two weeks for this.
● Perform movements, 2, 8, 10, 12, 13, and 20 from The top 20 twice each week for the next month of your practice. Perform all of The top 20 movements once each week during this time.
● Use the Image for each movement during two of your top 20 practices; use the Posy during the remaining one.

MBE   You have a strong mind and are probably very rational and logical. You most likely view your body in quite a practical way and are fairly relaxed about your size, shape and appearance. On the occasions when you fall ill (you are usually quite healthy) you slide into a mild depression. You should learn to trust your body a bit more than you do and you can do this by developing the links between your physical and emotional natures.

● Perform all of The basic 12 movements once each week throughout your practice.
● Become familiar with The top 20 movements by making the Voyages described in Chapter 5. Take one or two weeks for this.
● Perform movements 4, 7, 8, 12 and 14 of The top 20 twice each week for the next month of your practice. Perform all of The top 20 movements once each week during this time.
● Focus most closely on the Posy listed for each movement during your three top 20 practices. The comment listed after the number of each movement may help you get a better feel for the movement too.

MEB   You are also a rational, logical, possibly academic person — however much you may feel these qualities are disguised in you. It is possible that you sometimes get overwhelmed with feelings, perhaps finding it difficult to express yourself at these times. Your body is there for you when you remember it, which isn't often as your life tends to centre on your thoughts and feelings. So you will benefit from considering your body a bit more. These movements should provide fairly immediate help.

● Perform all of The basic 12 movements once each week throughout your practice.
● Become familiar with The top 20 movements by making the Voyages described in Chapter 5. Take one or two weeks for this.
● Perform movements, 1, 4, 7, 14, 19, and 20 of The top 20 twice each week for the next month of your practice. Perform all of The top 20 movements once each week during this time.

- Work on the details of your movements to achieve as much correctness as you can, then work to perform them gracefully. Consider the Posy for each movement as you perform it.

EBM You tend to live according to your 'heart': your feelings, intuitions and moods. This can be inconvenient in times or situations that don't allow your particular brand of spontaneity. You tend towards good health, although if you are slightly under the weather you find it difficult to feel motivated. You don't like too much brain work because you usually find it depressing or tiring or just too much effort. So you will benefit from working with co-ordination and movements that challenge your mental output. But don't worry, this is fun too!

- Perform all The basic 12 movements once each week throughout your practice.
- Become familiar with The top 20 movements by making the Voyages described in Chapter 5. Take one or two weeks for this.
- Perform movements, 3, 7, 9, 11, 14 and 20 of The top 20 twice each week for the next month of your practice. Perform all of The top 20 movements once each week during this time.
- Hold the Image given in your mind while you perform each movement. You will benefit from frequent repetition of the movements while concentrating on this image.

EMB You experience very strong feelings and then proceed to battle with them by insisting that they produce logical and rational reasons for being there. You may have a temper or, at least, suffer from flashes of acute frustration, impatience or intolerance. Your body takes the brunt of your dis-ease at these times by getting headaches, a nervous stomach or a tremendous sense of fatigue. You will benefit from physical challenge that holds your concentration so you will cope well with fairly complex movements — provided you allow yourself a bit of time to learn them.

- Perform all of The basic 12 movements once each week throughout your practice.
- Become familiar with The top 20 movements by making the Voyages described in Chapter 5. Take one or two weeks for this.
- Perform movements, 1, 5, 7, 14, 15-19 and 20 of The top 20 twice each week for the next month of your practice. (Movements 15-19 should be learned separately and then performed in sequence to create a complex, diagonal movement across the floor. Both arms will be moving as you step.) Perform *all* of The top 20 movements once each week during this time.
- Work most diligently on the details of your movements, however much you would like to say 'that'll do' to yourself. Chapter 6 has some useful techniques for improving your control of detail. Consider the Image given for each movement if your concentration starts to wander.

You will notice that the first four to six weeks of your practice are given special attention. The reason is that this period of time is used to become familiar with the movements and to acquire a sense of your own personal balance. This initial period of practice will also reveal the quality of communication that already exists between your physical, mental and emotional natures. Over this time you will stimulate the less powerful aspects of your personality so that balance, communication and progress will ensue without you having to force them.

After this time, assuming you have performed your schedule of movements as suggested, you may use the following, standard schedule:

- Perform The basic 12 once each week to give a constant foundation to your practice. You may, if you like, reassess yourself on occasion to see if your score, and therefore your code, has changed. A change in your code is quite likely and very interesting but not as important as your *initial* code. (If you have stopped your movement practice for a period of time, however, your new score will be as important as your initial score.) The basic 12 movements give you a picture of your present state of balance; they provide your starting point for your Movement Design practice.
- Perform The top 20 movements three times each week. Do all 20 if you can. If that is not possible, then select your favourites and those you find most challenging. The top 20 maintain balance and progress in your personality.
- Focus on the Image for one of your weekly top 20 practices; on the Posy for another, and on the physical detail of your movements for the third weekly practice.
- It is possible to perform all of your movements in 10 to 15 minutes. Or you may perform them over 30 to 40 minutes. It's your choice.
- You may perform them fast or slow, to music or in silence, in company or by yourself.
- You may laugh or remain serious.

41

- You may perform the movements in any order and repeat any of them any number of times.
- You may, in fact, design your own sequences to combine these movements in an order and in a form most pleasureable and appropriate to you.
- The last two chapters in this book will suggest some additional movements suitable for the particular needs and developments your body may display. You may incorporate any of these movements into your weekly practice or you may choose to perform them only as and when you feel they are necessary to your health.

Please continue your use of the Change games from Chapter 2 as you learn The basic 12 movements. Give yourself as much time as you like to become familiar with both the games and the movements. Stay relaxed.

Chapter 4
Movement Design explained

I began, many years ago, a private pursuit — a train of thought. I wanted to understand the mechanisms, if there were any, of personal and human progress because it seemed to me that progress was a challenge set especially for people. We — of all animal life— seemed perpetually to create opportunities and dilemmas that thrust us backwards or forwards into yet more opportunity and dilemma. I felt that our strength and our only security lay in our ability to cause — and accept — the progressive change that grew out of these opportunities.

The concept of progress did not become formal until the 16th and 17th centuries. Before that time, many people — Aristotle for one — thought that all there was to be known was already known, so intellectual efforts were therefore aimed at emulating earlier cultures and social systems. But, while most people did the emulating, some people went ahead and did original things such as inventing the printing press, gunpowder and navigational instruments. Through these people progress was confirmed as fact and made formal as a concept. These people had experienced something, something that made them create change.

It was this thing that I found alluring. I wanted to know precisely how a person could be at one place in their development one moment, and the next have travelled incredible distances within their own potential. I wanted to find that split second of change and look at it. I wanted to know why it came about at all.

I had no doubts that progress existed: I had seen it in others and I had even felt it in myself. I wanted to communicate to others a complete understanding of our human ability to create and endure changes that lead to progress, but first I had to find a starting point.

I began my pursuit from the observation that we are each a composite of body, mind and emotion. I strongly suspected that body, mind and emotion work together to create all that is human about us, that they are inextricably linked, that they are, and always have been, of equal importance to our makeup, and that our emphasis or de-emphasis of one or the other of them determines our health, our history, our direction, our rate of progress and the quality of our lives. In the years I spent developing the Movement Design concept, I tested and investigated these ideas and then searched for a means of communicating my findings.

I had a strong feeling that progress, or the potential for it, was contained within each one of us, that if it manifested as a social or cultural phenomenon, then that was by the force of personality — whether of one person or many. So, I needed to know the personality in its fundamental form.

Personality is the quality contained within the condition of being a person. That is rather a mouthful, but it is also very apt. A person several yards from you in a crowd is only a person. That same person talking with you over coffee is a personality: the person has come to life. They are distinctive, individual and you are able to be a personality in return, to them. The manifestation of personality, of this quality, and the communication of it occurs in three modes: physical, mental and emotional. I could find no more. Every additional or alternative mode I came up with turned out to be, in fact, a subset of one of those three. So I needed, next, to look at each of these three modes in turn.

I looked first at emotion and thought that I might find my answers almost before I started. I was fairly sure that studying emotion would reveal the mechanisms I sought, but I found, and still find, the subject nearly dead. The emotional aspect of the personality is currently so neglected and underrated as to cause embarrassment and fear at simple discussion of it. Socially and culturally it seems present only in art and in newspapers. In the latter, it is brandished as a derogation of the person or subject in question. How many times have you read the word 'emotive' in the context of 'worse-than-valueless'?

Emotion in a medical sense usually means that heads shake from side to side 'Poor fellow, lost his job too. Emotional troubles.' Emotion appeared to be problematical. No one would talk to me about it, yet I still felt that it was an essential and powerful component of personality. I knew that its position within us was pivotal but I could arrive at no exploration of it that could be clearly and easily communicated. I could find no method, accessible to a great variety of people, that resulted in a reawakening of emotional comprehension and fluency. I could not see any overt connection between emotion and human progress.

I looked next at the mind and I admit I did this with wariness. The mind has held our attention for hundreds of years, in which time it has become dominant and masterful. My wariness was based on the great disparity between the sheer weight of public belief about the mind and my own seemingly solitary suspicions about it. While it has accounted for much social and cultural reformation and while it has been proffered as the difference between animals and humankind, I found that it was also the source of much that was erroneous and damaging to us. I did not see it as the seat of progress, although it had often been purported as such. I did not find it all-powerful or conclusively human. Instead, I found the mind extravagant and somewhat rampant.

I observed that, in social and historical terms, complete trust had been placed in the mind. It had been given unrestrained access to our lives — in both a personal and cultural sense. I saw that its own nature prevented it from modifying these bequests in the slightest and the result, I perceived, was one of dominance causing narrowness. I saw the mind depriving itself of input from anything other than more mind. I could not believe that this situation was one that could sustain progress, nor, I concluded, was it a situation that could initiate it.

The body drew my attention finally. I studied anatomy and physiology, subscribed to medical journals and acquainted myself with the many branches of modern medical practice. I observed and then sampled various forms of fitness training, studied movement and dance, watched myself and others

in illness and health and read what I could find about the history of the human body. I realized, as a result, that the body is, and for some time has been, abused. Abused by ourselves, abused by others, abused in health and illness. The body was not the cornerstone of human progress I was seeking. It was, in fact, treated more like a millstone around the neck of human progress. We still clothed the body in remnants of shame and privacy and punishment, we still felt uneasy with the animal nature that partly defined it and we seemed still to hold a literal view of the body, one that diminished our responsibility for it and couched its functions in mechanical terms.

The body is often referred to as a machine, yet I could find little that was mechanical about it. I sought mechanisms. I looked for the spark, the gearing, that would be the source of motion, of progress, but I observed only a listlessness in the body.

At this point I paused. This was all we had. This was the sum of personal attributes, so far as I knew. I spent some time then playing with synonym: sameness in a different guise. I read some philosophies and listened to some religions to discover their format and their approach to the personality. I even looked towards the collection of therapies that have appeared in abundance since the 1960s. These were very current and broadly accepted. They dealt with everything I had looked at — body, mind and emotion — in a way that I had never considered and they seemed very popular. But none of these therapies were correct, not even in their own terms. None was entire enough.

True therapy is healing, but I found none of those that I studied was healthy, let alone healing. These therapies placed blame, were neither positive nor progressive. They were based upon one portion of the personality — say, for instance, emotion — that would in the course of therapy become the scapegoat for all personal problems and errors. The therapy used this portion, placed blame upon it and seemed then to batter it into numbness. Emotional therapy involved, to me, emotional suicide. Mental therapy seemed, to me, mental trauma and vindictiveness. Physical therapy appeared, to me, little short of brutality.

I observed that most therapies gave an outlet, a focus, for a great many people. But I did not observe that the therapies allowed progress and in some cases I observed that they actually prevented progress or, worse, caused retrogression. I knew then that therapy was nearly the antithesis of what I sought and what I hoped to establish.

At approximately this time, I was operated on to remedy the effects of what had, apparently, been a mild case of polio contracted in my early youth. One foot had gradually splayed until, at the time of the operation, it was about six inches wide. Walking had become an extremely painful experience, one that I was increasingly forced to avoid, and my life seemed to narrow at the same rate as my foot broadened.

Thankfully, the operation was successful, but I spent one year recovering from it. That whole year was a deeply unhappy one for me. It was also one of the greatest personal opportunities I have ever had.

During that year I was freed from the many tasks and demands that required a mobility I didn't possess. Of course, I didn't see it as freedom immediately, I saw it as handicap, I felt temporarily disconnected from others and from the buzz of life around me. I felt isolated and devalued, but worst of all, I felt stopped, as though I had ground to a halt . . . and I had. I experienced not only physical immobility but personal immobility.

My lifeline was, as I am certain it has been for thousands of other people, within myself. I began to notice more about the people near me. I began projects and read books that I had always meant to get around to and I was able to pursue trains of thought that had previously been continually interrupted — and therefore abbreviated — by the demands of a normal, mobile routine.

Very shortly, I picked up the strands of my search for the mechanics of human progress and suddenly I saw what I had been unable to see before. Suddenly the whole panoply of human progress glistened at me out of my notebooks and scribblings.

I saw that the mechanism of progress is relationship — intrapersonal relationship, that is, relationship within ourselves of the three aspects of the personality. I saw that progress is more to do with the links between body, mind and emotion than it is to do with body, mind and emotion themselves. And more.

I saw that progress is either personal or cultural. That is, we may experience progress in and for ourselves but that that progress need have nothing to do with our culture. Or, we may be part of cultural progress, yet that progress need have nothing to do with our own intimate progress. We may experience both simultaneously, but the two occur on different time scales.

In cultural progress the relationships between body, mind and emotion manifest themselves over long periods of time using the bodies, minds and emotions of the people who sustain the culture. Personal progress on a massive scale, or on a smaller scale over a long period of time, has the potential to instigate cultural — even world — progress. Cultural progress is an emergence or evolution, often outliving generations of people.

Personal progress occurs only to the individual, no matter to what degree they are affected by their culture. Personal progress occurs only when the links between body, mind and emotion are functioning — because relationship, that thing essential to progress, is communicated along these links. Recall the spinning triangle from Chapter 3, the internal Meeting 4. In that example communication inspired a relationship that produced balance, a relationship that linked all three aspects of the personality and created, therefore, a state of progress for the individual. Personal progress may be an undertaking or it may be in the nature of an inspiration. It may be cultivated over a period of time or it may come upon one in a flash.

Once I had realized that relationship was the mechanism of progress, I was able to see more clearly the importance of various characteristics within the natures of body, mind and emotion. I was, at this time, still in plaster, still using crutches and still very depleted in my physical resources, but I was very eager and energetic in my thoughts and observations. In order to communicate progress, in order to show others how they might spark it in themselves, I needed to know and understand the relationships that linked body, mind and emotion together within each person. I needed to be able to speak them, demonstrate them if necessary and certainly reveal them in others. So, I began to experiment on myself.

A summary of these experiments will suffice here. They were based on co-ordination, visualization, expressive techniques, hand movements, rhythm, aural preferences, sleeping postures, silence, breathing, balance, muscular tension, positive thinking, use of language, symbol and medium and they continued for a further three years.

At the end of that time I taught the first classes in Movement Design. It wasn't called that at first, but the formula was the same in that first communication as it is now.

Movement Design is a system that is founded on uniqueness and personality. It was begun as a celebration of life and movement and it continues this celebration by creating opportunities for health, communication and personal progress in the individuals who practice it.

I arrived at movement as the best means of establishing, communicating and maintaining the intrapersonal relationships that allow progress. This was the only activity that spanned all of history, all of human experience and that, although obviously physical, used body, mind and emotion simultaneously and in equal portions. I then developed movements and movement sequences that could be greatly altered in their dynamics. I needed movements that could be designed to suit whoever used them — no matter what their age, mobility, size, or state of health.

I very much wanted these movements to be a pleasure to perform, yet they had to achieve the goals I planned for them. Each movement had to create or reiterate awareness within the person, begin or be part of a process of change and have the potential to become habitual.

In Chapter 3 you learned 12 movements that enable your body to give voice to the present state of balance within your personality. Although a great many other people have learned and practised these very same movements, they are different for each person and that is as it should be. If you perform the movements in your own way, they will work for you in a manner, and at a pace, appropriate to you. Movement Design is for you, it is fun and it is successful.

There are three fundamental stages in Movement Design:

- The creation of movements
- The practice of these movements
- The use of these movements to establish intra-personal relationship and thereby initiate progress

Each of these stages have criteria to fulfill and these are outlined below.

The creation of movements

Balance

All the movements in the Movement Design repertoire must be balanced in their use of body, mind and emotion. In other words, they must give equal importance to each of these aspects of your personality. How is that possible when movement makes such obvious use of the body? Well, firstly, the movements, although simple, require that you think, they are intellectually challenging. The movements also cause you to experience emotion while performing them. The emotions will be both obvious and subtle, positive and negative.

Ensuring that the movements are balanced in this way further ensures that your practice will be ever changing in its effects. You may repeat these movements every day for the rest of your life, and they will always feel different because, if one single thing in your life changes from one day to the next — and it always does — then so will your practice.

Appropriateness

Every movement included in the Movement Design repertoire must be made appropriate to the person performing it. Appropriate to you: your shape, size and physical condition, your circumstances, environment and level of commitment, appropriate to your needs and aspirations, your unique nature.

That is a giant task and Movement Design can't do it alone. You must become partly responsible because only you know your body entirely. In Chapter 2, you confronted a lot of home truths about yourself simply by observing them. That was your starting point and you must always start by observing where you are.

Movements that are created to be appropriate to you in a physical sense are more likely to be suited to your mental and emotional natures as well. Appropriate movements will parent thoughts and feelings that support balance, enhance your sense of self and reiterate your uniqueness.

Safe, simple and successful

Movement Design forbids pain, there is enough of that in the world already. It forbids the brutality implicit in ignoring signals from body, mind or emotion. If a movement is balanced in its use of body, mind and emotion and if that same movement is appropriate to the individual and his or her many needs, then it is extremely unlikely that the movement would ever be dangerous or unsafe. A safe and comfortable movement allows the mind and emotions to remain in proportion to the body. This same proportion keeps the movement simple or accessible so that even the most 'unphysical' person may perform it. Safe and simple movements are easily repeated and, in terms of Movement Design, that makes them successful. If you are able to repeat these movements with ease then you will derive as much from them as it is possible to derive, in physical, mental and emotional senses.

Progressive

The final criterion of the creation of Movement Design movements is that they be progressive. They must enhance or instigate progress, development or growth in the person doing the moving.

Progress always starts with awareness and awareness is really a form of acknowledgement, an acceptance of some characteristic within yourself, a sort of 'OK, I admit it!' Awareness says, 'I know everything I do' it doesn't say, 'Everything I do is fine'. Movement Design uses movement to inspire your awareness of body, mind and emotion.

Progress builds upon itself when you set goals and employ process. Process is a joyous state. It means: purposefully undertaking a series of changes that you have directed towards progress of a given nature. Said another way, process is 'going for it' with a positive, determined and well-planned course of action.

Now you come to what is very like a paradox. Part of the progressive cycle is the formation of habits, but part of the retrogressive cycle is the formation of habits, too. How can you tell the difference?

Backtrack slightly to where we talked about awareness. If you are aware, then you know what habits you already possess and you may be further aware of which of those habits are 'bad'. Not all habits are bad, some are very good, indeed, some are essential. Habits are the nearest you get to running on automatic: without thought, without feeling, with little sensation. Habits free you from reconsidering actions and thoughts and feelings that are working just fine. Therefore, 'good' habits are stabilizing, they support progress and engender self-trust. Good habits are those that you create for yourself out of consideration for yourself — out of awareness. Bad habits create inertia and leave you in a rut — they are retrogressive.

Movements are progressive if they grow out of awareness, employ process and arrive at habitual use of movement to maintain or secure the progress gained.

The practice of movement

Maintenance

After their careful creation, these movements are practiced while maintaining the criteria outlined above. Each movement must remain balanced, appropriate, safe, simple and progressive during every practice. If these criteria are truly maintained, then there need be no other form of monitoring utilized for the purely physical aspect of Movement Design.

Mental images and attitudes reformed

Assuming you acquire some degree of ease with many of the movements, this point in your practice will require you to observe your mental images and attitudes — as you did in Chapter 2. Based on the awareness gained through observation you may reform your mental images and attitudes.

Mental images are, like the movements, at their best when they are appropriate and progressive. In order to give yourself the best of your mind, you must start from where you are and set about changing what needs changing.

Emotional patterns reformed

Emotion is full of bad habits and, somehow, those that aren't bad seem just too quiet to make much difference in the normal run of things. In this part of the practice you allow an equal voice to all of your emotional patterns but first you watch. Refer to Chapter 2 again to remind yourself how to watch your emotions. Then reform your emotional habits and patterns by simply selecting those you want to keep. Continuous selection of those patterns while reinforcing them through movement will ensure that you retain good emotional habits.

Discrepancy between awareness and goals

In the Movement Design practice you continually

observe your own position, continually seek balance and appropriateness in it and, as a result, are ensured of both safety and progress. This is true for each of the physical, mental and emotional elements of the practice. You have done a lot of observation and, by now, may have a fairly clear understanding of these three aspects of your personality. Now you can really get down to using that understanding.

'Draw' two blueprints each for body, mind and emotion. On the first of each, outline what you possess in that part of your personality. On the second, outline what you hope to possess. Now compare them. This part of Movement Design practice is an observance of the discrepancy between awareness and goals, the discrepancy between what you know you are and what you hope to become.

Discrepancy is a catalyst. It is an incentive to change, to create, to act. There will always be discrepancy between your awareness and your goals. Your aim must be to minimize this discrepancy and thereby achieve the maximum progress, the most positive change, the most appropriate life for yourself.

Movements to establish relationship

In the final stage of the Movement Design practice you assign specific movements and body locations to mind and emotion.

Locating mind in the body

Certain places in and certain movements of the body have a fairly direct access to the mind. These are approximately the same for most people. However, it is necessary for you to experience these locations and movements for yourself. (See Chapter 5.)

Locating emotion in the body

There are definite places in and movements of the body that pertain specifically to emotion. These movements and locations might be difficult to find at first, but they are quite unforgettable once you do find them. They may be easily experienced after some guidance. (See Chapter 5.)

Tracing the connections

Have you ever played 'dot-to-dot' games? You are given a page full of numbered dots that you then join up with lines resulting in a picture. Similarly here. Your body is dotted with places that are particularly responsive to mind or to emotion. It is for you to connect each set of 'dots' so that you complete a picture of your mind/body relationship and a picture of your emotion/body relationship. But what about the mind/emotion relationship?

Your task in this stage of Movement Design is to locate mind and emotion in the body, to join the lines, make the connections, allow the relationships that follow. Then, to make the final, vivifying link you lay these two dot-to-dot pictures one over the other. Still in this analogy, draw a third set of lines. This time connect the first mind dot with the first emotion dot, then the first emotion dot with the second mind dot, on to the second emotion dot, from there to the third mind dot, and so on.

Suddenly your drawing is three-dimensional. Suddenly you are looking at a picture of your personality. You have completed the triangle, the internal Meeting 4, and have created balance because once the third and final connections are made, the picture comes to life, it moves and then so do you.

The culmination of your Movement Design practice is your ability to trace, with understanding, the final, vital picture of yourself by moving through all of these connections. You trace links and create relationship.

Do this as you feel. Slowly, at high speed, joyously, pensively, in health or illness, but always with awareness. Always with the knowledge that you are establishing intrapersonal relationships that will create balance, health, intelligence, wisdom and, of course, progress.

Chapter 5
Voyages round your body

You have probably played this game, either as an adult or as a very young child just learning to talk. The adult says, 'nose' and the young child puts its hand on its nose. Then the adult says 'mouth' and the young child puts its hand on its mouth and so on. If the child makes an error, putting hand to eye when the adult says 'ear', then the adult laughs and corrects the child by repeating the word 'ear' and holding the child's hand on its ear. It is a fun game for both and a very important one.

You learn about your body by using your body. The more you use it, and the more varied its use, the greater becomes your knowledge and the more thorough and considerate your use of it. You can develop a very detailed understanding of your body and its functions and arrive at a deep awareness of it by discovering, for yourself, its features and capabilities. You can study your own anatomy — the way you see it — from within yourself.

Knowing your anatomy from the inside will bring you greater health, greater control and greater enjoyment in your life because truly knowing your own anatomy creates a turning point in your treatment of yourself. On one side of that point, you continue with the conventions and policies given to you years ago. On the other side of that point, you invite appropriateness into your body, and your life. Learning from the inside is rather the opposite of what you are taught to expect from a study of anatomy, in which it is normal for others to tell you how you function, how your body feels, what it looks like, in which it is others who define and illustrate

your parameters of wellness and illness, in which others use a series of charts and diagrams to depict a standard for your bones, your muscles, your nerves.

Your inside knowledge of your anatomy is worth much more than these. Your intimate understanding and awareness tells you the truth about your body without requiring illustrations and textbooks and fluent Latin. In order to know your own anatomy you need only learn it for yourself by moving through it.

The top 20 movements on page 52 are selected to help you begin your exploration of your own physical anatomy. As you perform them, imagine that your movements are voyages drawn out on a map. Imagine that every sensation, every surprise or realization, every balance or stretch, is a landmark on that map. Perform all 20 movements as best you can (there are instructions to help you with the details of your practice), then repeat the movements as though you were on a return journey: stop at every feature, every sensation, every landmark that you have previously positioned on your map of body, and place new landmarks as they happen.

These movements trace your physical anatomy. They are a journey that lets you renew contact with areas of body, physical sensations and styles of movement that you may not have experienced for a very long time — or ever before. These movements are a voyage that you may take over and over again, a map that you may unfold or alter at any time, throughout your life.

Voyage 2

When you have become familiar with the Top 20 movements, add another dimension to your map. Set out on a new voyage to investigate the qualities and characteristics of each landmark and feature marked on the map of your physical anatomy. This is a voyage to learn your own mind.

Your mind manifests itself in the form of rules and patterns and memories that affect the function and health of your body. Because your mind complies so well to its own rules and patterns, it is quite easy to trace its anatomy. Mental anatomy comprises thought, reason, logic, rationale and the landmarks that these qualities create within you as a physical being. Your mental anatomy adheres to your physical anatomy, the two being inseparable except as ideas. Where the body describes the routes on the map of your voyage, the mind describes the terrain — the valleys and peaks of your personal anatomy.

When the two voyages are merged into one map, a straight route over your physical map may, for instance, become a straight but sloping trek across your mental map. Your mental anatomy exerts a very powerful effect on the quality of the movements you perform because, in applying its rules and patterns and memories to your body, it induces focus and concentration. Your entire personality becomes stronger as a result.

Repeat The top 20 movements, but now trace your mental anatomy by considering the Image suggested at the bottom of each page. Hold this image in your mind while you perform each movement. It will help you to focus your mind into your body and will locate your mental processes into your movement.

Voyage 3

Your map, so far, shows landmarks and features from your physical anatomy, and has the heights and depths of your mental anatomy superimposed upon these landmarks. Now you may add the crucial details. This, the most subtle of all, is a voyage to map and explore your emotional anatomy.

Emotion translates, communicates and transcends. It mediates between the needs and activities of body and of mind, but emotion is also the factor in your personal anatomy that enables balance, wisdom, joy, despair, anger, success and all the other personal qualities that appear on your map.

Emotion lives within you, between your body and your mind. This is an emotional fact, a physical fact and a mental fact too. Emotion has locations within your body: there are physical venues for it. Emotion has locations within your mind: there are mental processes especially for conveying it.

Yet emotion remains just an ear and a voice. It remains invisible except for its effects and these are manifold because emotion is the life-force within every person. It is the source of motivation during all personal growth and change. Your emotional anatomy may be felt, like an electric current, and the results of its presence may be seen, as in health and love and conversation, but it is a difficult creature to find and become familiar with in its own form. Yet that is exactly what you must do.

Continue to repeat The top 20 movements, but now, as you perform them consider the emotional Posy suggested at the bottom of each page. A Posy is a sort of motto, a brief line or two to help convince your emotions of the sense within each movement. Each Posy will help you to locate emotion in your movement. As you perform the movement, do your utmost to *allow* the emotion that results. Simply take note of it with as little thought, or consideration for your body, as possible. If you feel a thought coming, pull away from it. If you feel a great deal of attentiveness towards your body, pull away from that too. Emotion lives somewhere between them. You must find it and feel it and gradually become familiar with it.

The final anatomical map

Do you remember that internal Meeting 4 described in Chapter 3? Your next endeavour must be to make each of your movements as balanced in their use of body, mind and emotion as was that internal meeting.

Your body, your mind and your emotions must be involved to an equal degree in the manufacture and outcome of each movement. Every movement must allow that split-second of exchange between body, mind and emotion that is necessary to incur balance.

In this final voyage, you move to trace the relationships between the three aspects of your personality. In this voyage you mark, not the physical, mental or emotional features, but the sparks that fly between them.

When you next perform your movements, do not dwell on the physical or the mental or the emotional elements involved in the movement, simply perform the movement with as much presence as you can muster. Be deeply involved in every minute detail, every breath, every stillness and balance without once considering any of it.

This may seem very like a paradox. Nevertheless, during this stage of your movement practice, be at once as vague and as present, as serious and as humorous, as cautious and as carefree as you can. Do not notice, do not think, do not feel, only move.

The top 20

MOVEMENT 1:
Use all of the space in front and above you.

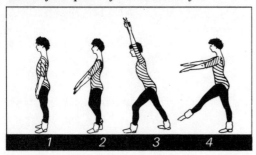

1 Stand tall with your feet hip-width apart, your arms relaxed at your sides. Keep your chin level and breathe.

2 Lift one heel away from the floor. Reach this leg behind you as you transfer your body-weight forwards onto the other leg. To counterbalance, raise both arms straight in front of you to about shoulder-height.

3 Keep your back leg stretched as you lower your toes then the heel onto the floor. Transfer nearly all your weight to your front leg as you bend it deeply at the knee. Both sets of toes should face forwards. At the same time, raise your arms above your head to create a straight line along the back of your body. Look to the floor in front of you.

4 Transfer your weight quickly onto your back leg by pushing your front toes firmly down towards the floor. Keep your front leg stretched in front of you at about hip-height. At the same time, lower your arms to shoulder-height. Repeat this movement using your other leg.

IMAGE

Support for your body does not come from the ground, it comes from above you. The lowest point of support for your body is in the sternum. This point is attached to the space and lightness above you. The rest of your body rests gently away from this point.

POSY

Belief in yourself is a 'yes' emotion. It does not mean telling lies about yourself, but does mean holding a positive attitude.

MOVEMENT 2:
Trace your centre. You have found it when you feel a tingle.

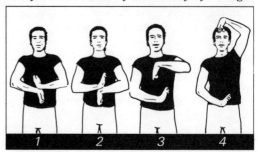

1 Stand or sit with your torso tall but relaxed. Bring your hands to navel-height and fold your fingers at the first and second knuckles to create a slight tension in the muscles of your hand. Now place one wrist close to your body in line with your centre, place the other wrist just in front of it.

2 Begin to rotate your hands at the wrists while, at the same time, circling your wrists around one another. Try this slow at first, then pick up speed. Circle in both directions keeping to your centre all the while.

3 Now place your wrists one above the other in line with your centre. Extend from the lower wrist and flex from the upper. Keeping these angles, pull the top wrist up, the bottom wrist down, to trace your centre.

4 When the top wrist has reached eye-level and the bottom wrist hip-level, reverse the angle of hand to wrist. Now re-trace your centre with the wrists moving in the opposite direction to the one they had been.

IMAGE

The final responsibility for your movement practice is yours — everything about it is of your choosing. That's how it can be made appropriate to you and what enables you to receive all the rewards that result.

POSY

Your centre is an emotion. It has a physical location compatible with the function of the body and it has intellectual acceptance because it creates symmetry. However strongly you feel your centre physically or mentally, it remains an emotion and is the seat of control and awareness.

The top 20

MOVEMENT 3:
When you cannot move forwards, move to each side.

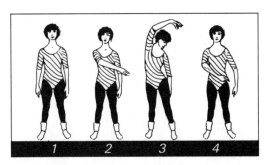

1 Stand tall with your feet shoulder-width apart, toes forwards. Allow your arms to hang freely at a slight distance from your sides. Keep your chin level and breathe easily.

2 Begin to raise one arm up and across your torso. Keep this movement in the arm alone, just for a moment. The hand is gently cupped with the thumb and forefinger pressed together.

3 Continue to raise this arm to above shoulder-level. At the same time, raise the heel of the foot opposite to the reaching arm. This will cause that hip to lift. Turn your face to look towards the hip.

4 Lower the lifted heel, turn your face forwards again and begin to lower the raised arm across your torso — all at once. Repeat this movement on the other side. You may speed it up once you become familiar with it.

MOVEMENT 4:
There is an arm's-length of space in all directions that you may carry with you at all times.

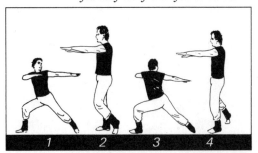

1 Step into a forward lunging position with both sets of toes facing forwards. At the same time, swing both arms to the same side as the back leg (see Figure 1 above). Keep your hands in line with your fore-arms and your arms at shoulder-level. Look back towards your outstretched arm.

2 Using the strength in both legs, pull yourself forwards to a standing position. Prepare to lunge forwards by bringing the back knee forwards. Swing your arms at shoulder-level straight out in front.

3 Step forwards into another deep lunge, on the opposite side to step 1. Swing your arms and turn your head at once. This may be a lyrical or a percussive, punchy movement.

4 Repeat the lunging movement as often as you like. Then finish by drawing into a balanced standing position with both arms stretched in front at shoulder-level. Feet are hip-width apart, toes facing forwards.

IMAGE

Movement includes stillness, as surely as music includes silence. Be as conscious and attentive in your stillness as you are in your movement.

IMAGE

Avoid haphazard movements: some movements may be damaging to you, some damage may be permanent. Thinking about your body as you move it allows you to respond in a safe, appropriate manner, one that enables progress and enjoyment.

POSY

Life is movement. Physical, mental and emotional movement. Life is an atmosphere of action, however subtle or austere.

POSY

Movement always has a motive: physical, mental or emotional. A movement is practical, expressive, communicative or a combination of these. Try to feel where the force, the motive, for each of your movements comes from.

MOVEMENT 5:
There is sharpness in every roundness.

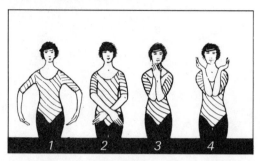

1 Stand or sit tall with your chin level and your shoulders relaxed. Hold your arms in a soft curve from shoulders to fingertips a little distance from your body — as though carrying a cushion under each arm.

2 Circle your arms forwards, moving from the shoulders, until your hands touch in front of you. Cross your wrists. Then stop the curving movement and, instead, pull your wrists sharply up towards your face. Keep your elbows low and near your body.

3 Bring your elbows together, then pull them close to the area of your navel. With the elbows tightly pressed together, your forearms will come together — look towards them. Slowly twist your fingers, hands and forearms outwards, from the elbows.

4 Keeping this twist, open the forearms but keep the elbows touching. Look forwards with your chin level. The final effect will be your hands and forearms framing your face. Breathe deeply.

MOVEMENT 6:
If you are forced to change direction, do it with grace and balance.

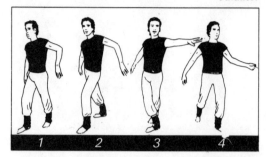

1 Standing, take a step forwards and, as you do so, lift the opposite arm up away from your side. This arm is bent at the elbow and still relaxed.

2 Take another step forwards and keep the same arm lifted and bending, even though you will feel imbalance. Exaggerate the sense of imbalance by stretching your arm out a little. To keep your balance, lean just your torso. Keep your pelvis central.

3 Continue to stretch your arm until it is straight. Instead of stepping forwards again, cross your leg in front and to the side (towards the stretched arm). Turn to look in this direction.

4 Put all your weight onto the leg that crossed. Turn your torso to line up with it and stretch the other leg behind you. The stretched arm may slowly relax down to your side. You have, in effect, made a right angle turn.

IMAGE

Allow fluctuations in the quality of your movements. To do otherwise would mean a regimentation of them. Fluctuations are often signs of impending progress or, as often, indicators of ailment, illness, fatigue or lack of attention. Treat fluctuations as opportunities.

POSY

The idea of separation between body, mind and emotion is not a fact — union is a fact. We are a union of those three parts; their separation is only possible as an idea.

IMAGE

Practice economy in your movements: use the least amount of effort, the least amount of muscular tension. Put your energy into making each movement as pleasurable and as beautiful as possible. When you think beautiful, you become beautiful.

POSY

Mistrust and reluctance are part of the 'no' emotion.

The top 20

MOVEMENT 7:
Great movement is always possible, even when your feet are stuck to the ground.

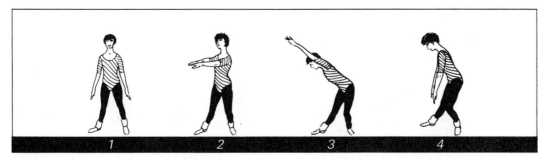

1 Stand tall with your feet shoulder-width apart. Keep one set of toes facing forwards, turn the others out at a right angle to the side. Let your arms hang straight but slightly lifted from your sides. Look forwards.

2 Begin to circle your arms and twist your torso at once so that you face towards your turned-out toes. As you do this begin to bend your knee (of the leg with toes facing forwards). Keep your arms straight as they circle.

3 Fold at the hips, stretch one arm back, one forwards. You will feel considerable stretch in your straight leg, and the need of strength in your folded leg. Hold this position briefly.

4 Maintain the position in your lower body and keep your back straight. Now lower both arms so that they reach towards your knees. Look down at your fingers. Breathe while you hold this briefly then step into a standing positon. Now try this movement on your other side.

IMAGE

When performing a movement that causes stretch in certain muscles, imagine a weight attached to those muscles. Now, whenever you do the movement, imagine the *weight* causes the stretch — don't feel that you have to do it. The result will be a more comfortable, more easily sustained and more successful stretch.

POSY

Enjoy as a child might the sensations of movement. Consider your ability to move a gift. Use it, and extend it if you can.

MOVEMENT 8:

There are many ways of seeing what is behind you.

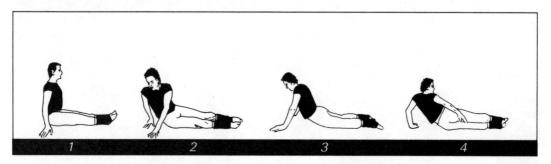

1   2   3   4

1 Sit as tall as you can on the floor. Stretch your legs straight out in front of you and place your hands beside you — just touching the floor.

2 Reach one arm across your body and at the same time roll to the opposite hip. Keep your torso as upright as possible as you begin this roll. Catch your body-weight with the crossing arm.

3 Continue to roll across the front of your pelvis. Support your upper body-weight with your arms and use the crossed arm to maintain the momentum of your roll. Keep your torso tall.

4 Come out of the roll on the other side of your body. Roll onto the other hip and use the other arm to push you upright into the tall sitting position once again. Pause and then repeat in the other direction.

IMAGE

If your body is rigid, your life will be rigid too. The combinations of joints, muscle, tendon and ligament in your body enable movement that is fluid, soft, elastic, flexible, powerful and resiliant. Think of how each of your movements combines joint with muscle to create mobility.

POSY

Spontaneity in your thoughts, actions and feelings allows a free translation of what is within you. It requires no skill but itself: indulge, permit, admit.

The top 20

MOVEMENT 9:

Function is sometimes better understood when you change your point of view.

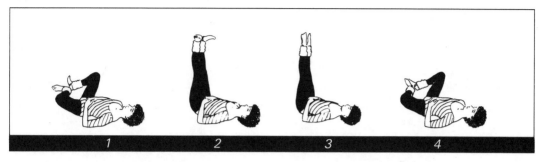

1   2   3   4

1 Lie flat on your back and cross your hands over your navel. Rest your elbows on the floor and tuck your chin comfortably close to your neck. Make certain that the back of your waist is on or near the floor. Now bring your knees up — one at a time — and allow them to relax wide apart. Flex your feet and press your heels together.

2 Keep your torso in the same position. Keep your heels firmly together. Now stretch your legs as far as you can directly up towards the ceiling.

3 Maintain this position but point your toes. Keep as much contact between the soles of your feet as you possibly can.

4 Keep the position of your feet the same but draw your knees back down and apart into the starting position. Try to keep your toes together as you do this. To repeat, flex your feet again.

IMAGE

Although your physical support comes from above you, your poor little feet take all of your living. Treat them well: step lightly onto them, make them as strong and flexible as you can, give them frequent massage. Your whole body will benefit from consideration given to your feet.

POSY

Dependence is a positive acceptance of relationship. It is a point of maturation beyond independence. This dependence is an emotional realization, one that amplifies the whole personality. It is delimiting rather than limiting.

The top 20

MOVEMENT 10:
The intersection of many lines creates energy, stillness and a link with infinity.

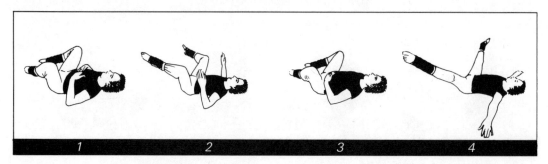

1	2	3	4

1 Lie flat on your back with your hands crossed over the base of your sternum. Keep your elbows away from your body and pressed onto the floor. Hold your chin comfortably close to your neck and press the back of your waist onto the floor. Now bring your knees up and relax them open. Keep your lower legs relaxed and your feet slightly pointed.

2 Now lift your forearms up to a right angle with the floor but keep your elbows down. At the same time, raise your lower legs to approximately right angles with your thighs. Stretch your toes as you do this.

3 Fold your lower legs back in towards your thighs again. Lower your forearms and place your hands over your navel. Double check that your knees are apart, your inner thigh muscles relaxed and stretched.

4 Stretch both arms out at shoulder level flat onto the floor. At the same time, stretch both lower legs straight out in line with the position of your thighs. If your legs do not stretch this much, then simply stretch them as far as you can without feeling trembles and without lifting the back of your waist from the floor. Hold briefly, breathe and then relax.

IMAGE

Feed your movements on breath and thought. Breath is most valuable in its exhalation, when it rids your body of lethargy, waste products, tension and fatigue. Thought supplies detailed guidelines to create a high-quality movement. Breath and thought together invite emotion into your movements.

POSY

When body, mind and emotion meet in equal parts there is control and awareness. When this happens, there is also the potential for correctness.

The top 20

MOVEMENT 11:
Angles are relationships, and they are either open or closed.

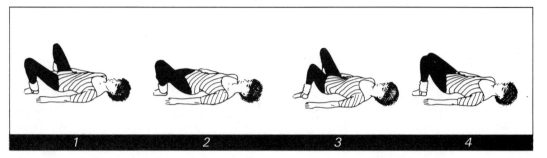

1 Lie on your back with your arms relaxed by your side. Keep your chin comfortably close to your neck and press the back of your waist onto the floor. Now fold your legs so that your feet are close to your body, about shoulder-width apart. Keep your knees apart also.

2 Lower one knee towards your opposite foot and rest there for two or three breaths in and out. Keep your other knee upright and your torso relaxed. You may need to increase the distance between your feet in the starting position in order to feel the full effect of this position.

3 Draw both knees upright and immediately reverse the movement, lowering your other knee towards its opposite foot. Hold for two or three breaths in and out.

4 Bring both knees to centre then allow them to move inwards to rest one against the other. Leave your feet in the starting position and rest there.

IMAGE

Experiencing the extremes of a movement or a position allows you to know the median. Explore these extremes in a gentle, positive way and, in each exploration, imagine a gently swinging pendulum or dial that eventually returns to its centre or beginning.

POSY

Thoughtlessness and trust in your body creates an opportunity for your emotional nature to mature.

The top 20

MOVEMENT 12:
A shape either hides or projects your motive.

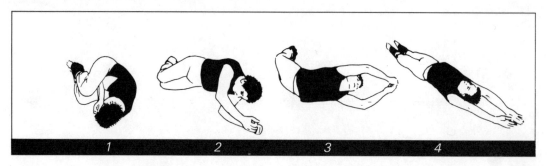

1 Lie on your side in what is commonly called a foetal position: tuck your knees up close to your body, fold your arms close to your chest, and curl your head inwards to round your back. Relax and breathe slowly.

2 Begin to open out into a stretch: unfold your legs, reach your arms up and forwards and lift your chin away from your chest.

3 Still resting on your side, extend both legs fully so that they arch behind you. Straighten your arms then reach them slightly behind you. Allow your back to arch deeply, point your toes and look up towards your hands. Breathe deeply at least one full breath.

4 Maintain this sense of stretch but eliminate the arch and roll onto your back. Close your eyes and hold this position for four breaths in and out.

IMAGE

Pain is the body's warning system. You should neither encourage it nor ignore it. Pushing yourself into pain or allowing it to continue discourages communication between the three aspects of your personality. It is not good for you on any level and does not speed progress of any sort.

POSY

Be gentle with yourself. Do not allow pain, discomfort or unhappiness in your movements. Try, instead, to enjoy the release of pain from your personality.

The top 20

MOVEMENT 13:
A curve is always part of a circumference.

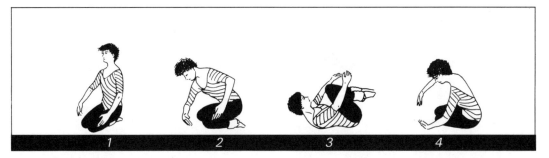

1 Sit on your heels with your back tall, arms resting by your sides.

2 Make a curve with one arm so that the palm of your hand faces up towards your face. At the same time, curl your body slightly forwards and lean to the side so that you are able to place some of your body-weight onto your curved arm.

3 Roll along your curved arm onto your side and immediately onto your back. Keep your knees close to your torso and begin to curve your other shoulder and arm a little.

4 Keep rolling, move onto the other side of your body and begin to roll along your other curved arm. Your momentum will help you to return to the upright position, sitting on your heels. If you sense a loss of momentum, simply straighten your arm slightly as you roll along it.

IMAGE

When you visualize a movement or position, compare it briefly with your actual performance of the movement or position. This comparison will provide you with a realistic view of what corrections need to be made. When you next perform the movement think all the while of the image you wish to fulfil. Your improvement will be rapid.

POSY

Pain is an emotion. It may emanate from any aspect of personality but is always translated into emotion, by emotion.

61

MOVEMENT 14:
Rhythm unites movement with stillness.

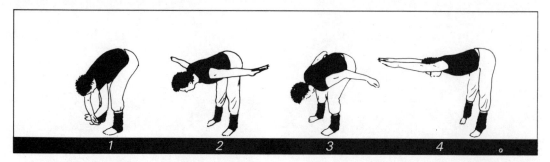

1 Curl forwards towards the floor (see Movement 7 of the Basic 12) and relax for one or two breaths. Now maintain the curled position, but swing your arms out to your sides and then across in front of your ankles. Try this three or four times to sense the rhythm of it.

2 Cross once again but, this time, as you swing your arms open to the side, straighten them and your legs at once. You may find it useful to look at one particular point on the floor in front of your feet. Hold this position for a few seconds then bend your knees and cross your arms once again.

3 Still in the curled position, swing your arms backwards and forwards by your side. Try this three or four times also to get the rhythm or bounce effect. The body remains curled and relaxed.

4 Swing your arms back but, this time, as they swing forwards, straighten and stretch them at shoulder level. Look towards your fingers. At the same time, straighten your legs and lift your heels off the floor. This is a very precarious balance to start with, but very stable after some practice.

IMAGE

Try not to be anxious or afraid when performing the movements. Some of them are unusual and may feel difficult or awkward at first. So, if you find yourself getting a little worked up, breathe out sharply, give your arms and hands a good shake and perform Movement 12 from Chapter 3. A good laugh will do wonders to relax you and put things into perspective again.

POSY

Focus and concentration are meetings of the emotional and mental aspects of your personality. Your gaze, the direction and placement of your vision, invites the physical into this union.

MOVEMENT 15:

Extending a limb may define or invade or dissect the space around you.

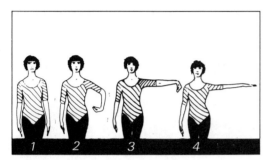

1 Stand or sit tall with your arms resting straight by your sides. In this movement, think specifically into one arm. Now think about the joints in that arm.

2 Fold your hand inwards towards your forearm and keep that tension while you reach your elbow out to your side. Bring your elbow up to as near shoulder-level as you can without loosening the tension in your wrist.

3 Straighten the whole of your arm out to the side at shoulder-level. Keep your hand flexed.

4 Keep your arm straight and then lift your hand until it is in line with your arm, palm facing downwards.

MOVEMENT 16:

Folding limbs are broken lines and create a withdrawal from the space around you.

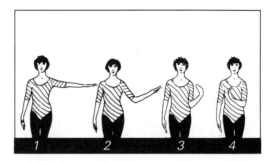

1 With your arm straight out to one side at shoulder-level (as Movement 15) simply turn your palm to face upwards.

2 Keep your palm facing up as you begin to pull your elbow in towards your body. Your hand may gradually fold in towards your forearm, too.

3 Pull your elbow deeply into your waist and, with your hand flexed inwards, begin to circle your forearm round in front of your body.

4 Relax your elbow from your waist only slightly as you complete the circular movement. Your hand is palm upwards in line with your other shoulder. You may perform this movement in sequence with Movement 15. Then repeat it using your other arm.

IMAGE

Attempt every movement on both sides of your body. For instance, if you are right-handed perform your movements with equal frequency and duration on your left side — and vice versa. If you avoid this challenge you diminish your movement repertoire by half.

POSY

Imitation of another takes you out of yourself and relieves the pressure of your own personality. It introduces you to empathy and observation.

IMAGE

Repetition of movements, if done intentionally and with awareness, stimulates communication between body, mind and emotion. Repetition helps to establish new habits, but this is only possible when you hold your attention on your body. If you let your attention slip off somewhere else, then you gain nothing.

POSY

Exaggeration is a way of arriving at the subtleness of an image, feeling or movement. You extend the possible to realize the actual.

MOVEMENT 17:
Your centre extends beyond you. It is much larger than your reach.

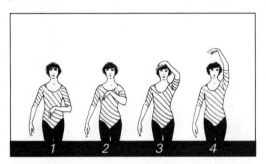

1 Stand or sit with one arm relaxed by your side, the other folded at the elbow with the forearm crossed in front of your waist, palm facing down. Think about your joints, in particular your wrist.

2 Raise your wrist to shoulder-level so that your hand is hanging down from it. Make this movement approximately in line with your centre.

3 Continue to raise your wrist to a height just above your eyes. The wrist is still leading, your hand is still hanging from it.

4 Complete this upward movement by stretching your arm fully above your head and in line with your centre. Keep your hand hanging from your wrist. Throughout, keep your chin level and look forwards.

MOVEMENT 18:
Your centre attaches most strongly to your body at your sternum.

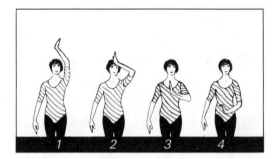

1 With your arm stretched fully over your head, pull the back of your hand towards your arm. Think of your wrist and keep your hand in this position as you begin to fold your arm at the elbow.

2 Bring your wrist down to a level just above your eyes. The wrist is still leading and your hand pulled tightly back. Keep your wrist moving along your centre.

3 Continue the downward movement of your wrist until it is about shoulder-level. Keep your elbow away from your body and keep looking forwards.

4 Complete the downward movement until your forearm has crossed in front of your waist. Keep your hand pulled tightly back to emphasize the sensation in your wrist. You may repeat this movement in sequence with Movement 17.

IMAGE
Your movement practice can be very social. Try joining in with someone else doing the movements. A very special atmosphere is often created: partly energetic, partly calm, always fun.

POSY
Anticipation of another's movements or behaviour is the beginning of kinship: you accept their personality and recognize its similarities with your own.

IMAGE
A movement starts in stillness and finishes in stillness. Your attention must endure for that entire period of time. Lack or loss of attention will delay or prevent the bodily awareness essential to health.

POSY
Acute bodily awareness creates an ability to transcend acute bodily awareness.

MOVEMENT 19:
Two lines at right angles always create a hidden diagonal.

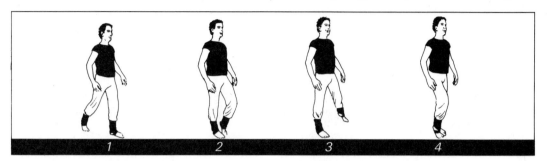

1 Stand tall with your arms relaxed by your sides. Look directly forwards with your chin level as you take one step backwards. Ensure that you step straight behind you.

2 As you transfer your weight onto the backwards-reaching leg, pull the front heel back to touch the side of your ankle. Keep your heel lifted and pause briefly in this position.

3 Now stretch the leg with the lifted heel in a straight line out to your side. Keep looking forwards as you transfer your weight onto this leg.

4 As you complete the weight transfer, pull your other leg close so that your ankles touch again. If you intend to repeat this movement, then keep your heel lifted. If you intend to stop here, then lower your heel into the floor.

Note: Movements 15 and 16 may be performed in sequence.

Movements 17 and 18 may be performed in sequence.

All four movements may be performed in sequence.

Movements 15, 16, 17 and 18 may be done in sequence while Movement 19 is also performed. Here's how:

Do step 1 of Movement 19 while performing Movement 17.

Do step 2 of Movement 19 while performing Movement 18.

Do step 3 of Movement 19 while performing Movement 15.

Do step 4 of Movement 19 while performing Movement 16.

Use the arm on the same side of the body as the leg that is stepping.

IMAGE

Everyone has physical limitations. Yours are unique to you and you would do well to view them as opportunities. They will help you to develop a personal and positive style of movement.

POSY

Expression is a clear and definite statement. Communication is an exchange: an imparting and a receiving. Expression is an opening to others but communication is relating to others. Communication is mature and progressive.

MOVEMENT 20:

Any part of your body may express the motivation for movement.

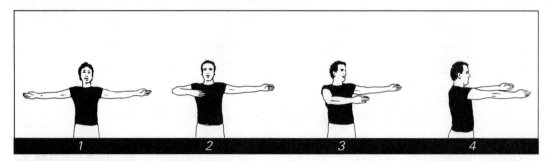

1 Stand tall with your feet shoulder-width apart, toes facing forwards. Stretch your arms at shoulder-level, straight out to your sides. Look forwards, keep your chin level and relax your neck. Breathe easily.

2 Maintain this position but fold one arm inwards at the elbow so that your hand touches the same shoulder.

3 Now pull that hand, at shoulder-level, across your chest and along your other arm. Follow the movement by turning your head and allowing your torso to twist. You will probably need to pivot slightly on your feet.

4 Continue to pull your hand along your other arm, always at shoulder-level. Allow your first, pulled, hand to reach beyond your second hand. Once the hand being pulled outreaches your other arm, begin to fold your (second) outreached arm at the elbow. Continue to pivot on your feet. This effectively reverses the movement and you will ultimately complete a 360° turn.

IMAGE

Memory makes use of your whole personality — body, mind and emotion. It is a question of translation: to remember a movement, translate it into its physical, mental and emotional components. When you wish to repeat the movement, translate its component parts back into a unit. Memorizing movements is a very pleasant challenge and improves your memory in other contexts too.

POSY

To unite your personality and to progress you must remain accessible to stimuli from others. This is your 'cycle of accessiblity': receive, interpret, remember, translate, act upon and receive again. If you break the cycle, you prevent unity and progress — you also remain inaccessible.

Chapter 6

The process of progress

Progress is the ultimate in appropriateness: if it isn't appropriate, then it isn't progress. Progress is always relative to you, it is any gain, improvement or forward movement measured from one hour ago or five years ago. It is the positive, active, effortful unfolding of your potential.

If you put effort into any part of your life then you will experience progress: it is a natural by-product of effort. For some people, the word 'effort' implies something fairly unpleasant, but effort includes even your favourite activities, it is part of every waking moment of your life.

On the back of every effort is a reward for making that effort in the first place. Reward is an acknowledgement, it is yours to enjoy, whatever form it takes. It feels good to be rewarded and that good feeling will make your next effort a little easier to initiate and sustain.

Effort and reward create a cycle: first you acknowledge that you put effort into your life, then you react to that effort by rewarding it, then you make certain you enjoy the reward because enjoyment will make your next effort a little easier to acknowledge. The spin-off to this cycle is change.

Change is another natural by-product of living and progress is simply a rather special form of change. It may be purposeful change that you cause to happen, it may be change that you simply shape as it comes your way or it may be the result of governing your reactions to change that has already happened. Progressive change is advancement and improvement: it can apply to your wage packet, your housing, your marriage, your reading list or your view of life. Progress is a repeated cycle of effort and reward creating changes that propel you into improvement.

Well, that's the theory, but what's so good about

it? What does it have to do with you, here and now?

As I've said, progress is going to happen to you anyway, whether you like it or not. It will either drag you forwards or accompany you forwards. It is up to you to determine which of these dynamics you'd rather live with. The former is reluctant, apathetic, and coercive, the latter is pleasant, positive and intentional. If you choose the former, then perhaps one day you will be dragged into a happy confrontation with intentional progress. If you choose the latter, then you may use this positive summary of intention to keep up the pace of your progress. It is easy to remember and a great aid, whether contemplating physical, mental or emotional progress:

Start from where you are
Look where you are going
Know when you are there

You know that progress results from effort and reward and you know that progress may be either intentional or coercive, but there are two components of progress that may enhance your personal rate of progress. They are process and habit.

Process

Process is a series of events: you are born, you live and then you die. You pick up an onion, then peel it, then you slice it. Events that are part of a process may occur over several years or within minutes of each other. They may occur with your involvement or they may 'happen to' you. You may perceive them as events that are part of a process or you may simply not notice them or their relationship with any other event.

If a series of events causes improvement or

advancement in you or what you are doing, then you are experiencing progress. Events are like stones across a stream: if you can move forwards from one to the other then you will eventually get to the other side, you will progress.

In your practice of Movement Design, each movement is an event. It can stand all by itself or it can become part of a series. You may perform the movement once in isolation, or you may perform it as part of a programme. To make your movements a process, you must start the movements, set goals for yourself (start from where you are, look where you are going) and then create movement events to link those two points together.

Process is also comprised of cycles. These are events that repeat to form a pattern. Cycles are very productive and comforting to take part in, they give meaning to each event and reiterate the goals and aims you have set for yourself — cycles keep your life moving.

A cycle starts with an event, is comprised of events and finishes with an event. A cycle runs its course and then repeats itself endlessly until a new event is introduced. In your Movement Design practice, a new event may be a sudden improvement in your co-ordination, it may be finding yourself able to do with ease a movement you previously found difficult or a realization that you are happier or more alert. Any of these would be a new event in the cycle you have established. When the new event occurs, or is introduced, you simply notice it and continue with your Movement Design programme. The programme remains the same but its character changes. You are repeating the same movement events in the same cycle but now your starting point is different because a new event has been introduced — you have improved, moved forwards, there is progress.

If you could draw this relationship between event and cycle, it would appear in two dimensions as a staircase. In three dimensions, as a spiral moving upwards and outwards.

Habit

The other component of progress that may assist you is habit. Habit is the Jekyll and Hyde of progress: you think you've got a good one then before you can blink it turns bad. The notion of habit is one that should keep you on your toes rather than leave you complacent. As discussed earlier, habit is the closest you get to running on automatic, but it is up to you to use that facility to your advantage and not allow

it to become a detrimental influence in your life. Here's how:

Firstly, become aware of your habits (take a look at Chapter 2 again to refresh your powers of awareness). They take many forms. You will notice that you have habits pertaining to what you eat, when you sleep, how you talk, where you shop and who you visit. You will also have habits in the way you move and think and feel. These latter examples are more difficult to become aware of because they are somehow less obvious and that is precisely why you should look at them. They are all the more powerful because they lie deeper within you and their subtlety is responsible for the firm grip they have on your life.

Secondly, make an assessment of your habits. Decide whether each is a habit of life-style or a habit of personality. For instance, working from nine to five, brushing your teeth twice a day and going out on Friday nights are all habits of life-style. Snapping at your spouse when you don't feel well, becoming aggressive when someone hurts your feelings and getting dewy-eyed over little babies are all habits of personality. These habits are not necessarily good or bad in themselves, but they are either good for you or bad for you. They will either stand in the way of your goals and your progress, or they will help you to achieve them.

So far, you have become aware of and assessed your habits. Now you must discriminate and select those you wish to retain and those you wish to eliminate from your life. Remember, the nature of habit is automation—not in the mechanical sense, but in the sense of functioning with the least amount of concern and attention. Progress is greatly enhanced if you are able to make habitual only those activities and characteristics that are appropriate to your personality, your life-style and your goals.

In your Movement Design practice, new habits are intentionally created to replace or undermine old or inappropriate habits. Habits that no longer have a place in your life are cluttering your practice or are opposing it. So, for instance, postural habits may be created that will free you from chronic backaches. Those backaches created habits that prevented you from enjoying your efforts and rewards, prevented you from progressing. They may have made you habitually decline to go on long walks with your family, or may have caused you to habitually concentrate less often on a hobby or study that you really enjoy. By finding, assessing and then altering the fundamental habit involved in this chain, you are able to open up your life and experience personal progress on many fronts.

The integrity of the body

Have you ever been out driving or walking and then, after a little while, realized that you are a mile or two down the road with no memory of how you got there? Something took over so that you were able to dream or think without even noticing that your body was still moving. If you were driving, your body actually performed all of the complex skills necessary to safe driving without you telling it to.

Many people who have found themselves in extreme danger have, in spite of great fatigue or injury, performed incredible bodily feats to save themselves or others. Most of these people report a narrowing of their perception to exclude all but the task in front of them. They realize afterwards that they don't recall making specific decisions but simply did what was necessary with no regard to the difficulty it might present.

Little children will sometimes, left to choose for themselves, feed predominantly on one food for weeks on end. They may then change to a completely new food preference with a seeming disregard for what had been the staple in their diet. Studies of this tendency have shown that the children are, in fact, selecting what is good for their body at that particular point in their development. Their preference is being dictated by their body's needs and not by parental or peer group pressure.

All the people in these examples are experiencing bodily integrity. Their bodies are responding to a situation without impaired or corrupted function. In these people the body is trusting itself completely, without any reservation whatsoever, to do what is most essential.

Your body has the same ability. Your body will respond in a similar way to meet all of its needs, but very few of us allow this to happen. Unless you are in a particularly relaxed or dangerous or uninhibited situation, you tend to interfere with your bodily signals. You think about them too much or attach emotional overtones to them that detract from the clarity and significance they originally had.

Your body is entire. It has a knowledge of itself that will maximize your health and safety and level of vitality. During your Movement Design practice, the 'voice' from your body will speak clearly and forcefully concerning all its many needs and characteristics. It will be left to you to 'listen' to these messages and respond to them.

For instance, if your body tells you that a movement should be left out of today's practice then leave it out! Don't think about it and say to yourself, 'Well, I might as well do it. There's really no reason why I shouldn't.' And don't bully yourself with 'I'm not going to slow down just because I don't feel like working so hard.' Both attitudes are denying your body's right to declare its needs, both are inappropriate to you and both are retrogressive.

Your body speaks through pain, discomfort, reluctance and fatigue. Through these it asks you to recognize its needs and modify your actions. It is for you to trust your body, to have confidence in those signals. You will slowly gain this trust and confidence while practicing your movements and you will compound that confidence once you find your body repaying your trust with physical delight, exuberance and wellness.

The mind's eye

When I was 14, I joined a diving club — because I was terrified of diving! I was a good swimmer, but every time I stood more than a short distance above the water I got a bit shaky. Well, I never excelled at diving, but I got over my fear of it and I did that by using the very old, very simple technique of imagination. Today it is called visualization.

An image is a mental picture and your body is one of the easier mental pictures for you to make and to keep hold of.

Try it now:

Imagine yourself standing or sitting in a park. Don't look at the park, just 'look' at you. Now imagine yourself talking with a friend. Picture both yourself and your friend in your imagination. There is nothing difficult or unusual about this at all, you probably use your imagination in this way every day, but when you are trying to improve or progress you may employ your imagination a little more emphatically. In your Movement Design practice there are two steps in using your 'mind's eye' to its greatest effect.

Making films

As a first step, do all your movements in your head. You may be in the bath, on the bus, at the beach, but all the while make a mental film of yourself doing a particular movement. 'Roll' the film, over and over again, from beginning to end. Use all of the technology of the film industry to help you: freeze frame, rewind, slow motion, fast forward, pause. Study the film in this way until you have memorized the movement. Then go try performing the movement yourself.

How to be the most beautiful you

Now go and stretch out on the beach again and roll the mental film once more, but, this time, touch up each frame of the film so that every detail of you, and the movement, is perfect. Take it to an extreme (in your head) if you like: polish your teeth and groom your toe-nails. The point is to make each image within that film as beautiful as possible. Imagine that you are the most beautiful diver or dancer or mover in the world. Infuse a special quality into each action and pose. Make certain that charisma simply oozes from every frame. When you have made your mental film as over-the-top perfect as you can, go and perform the movement yourself.

Your mind excells at a challenge of this sort. Not only does the technique work wonderfully at improving your movements, it also makes tremendous fun out of them. The whole experience becomes game-like and joyful. It is made less stressful than if you simply learned the movement through sheer grind. A word of caution, however, don't settle for anything less than beautiful when you imagine yourself doing that movement. You want to do your best so put everything into the image you hold inside your head. It will support you during your entire practice so that you receive as much from the movement as you possibly can.

All strings attached

Do you recall ever receiving a gift from someone but feeling that they weren't really there in the giving? You had the thing, the gift, but there didn't seem to be any sense of the other person in it. As a result, both the gift and the occasion are remembered as drab or perhaps a little sad.

So, with any activity or involvement, you may be either fully present or somewhere on the outer limits of the experience. There are only the two options and both are emotional statements and prerequisites. The former is an emotional 'yes' and invites opportunity, potential and progress; the latter is an emotional 'no' and refuses opportunity, potential and progress. An emotional 'yes' is a summary of every positive feeling in your life; an emotional 'no' is a distillation of every negative or nondescript sensation that intrudes upon your life.

Yes and no constitute your emotional repertoire. Within these two categories are numerous subtleties and specifics, but every emotional response you have emanates from one of these categories and indicates either your complete presence or absence from a particular moment.

In your Movement Design practice you may be fully present during each movement or you may keep part of your attention elsewhere. The first is an emotional 'yes', the second is an emotional 'no'. The first allows progress, enjoyment, health and confidence, the second allows boredom, stress, loss of reward and lack of progress.

Performing your movements with your total presence requires only ten seconds of your attention. It does not require an empty room in a quiet house in the middle of nowhere. You can give full attention to a movement and then turn to stir the spaghetti, if you like. Indeed, these movements are best done within the context of the rest of your life because the progress you are achieving is progress in the whole of your life. Performing the movements with an emotional 'yes' means that you are backing up your actions, you are committing yourself to your own potential, you are saying 'all strings attached' instead of 'no strings attached'.

Progress is a process of growth, during which you rely on events and cycles and habits. Progress asks that you move your body and trust it, that you use your mind to create mental images that sustain that trust and confidence. Progress asks that you support your physical and mental input into each experience by being there, by attaching yourself fully to every moment of your life, by saying 'yes' to the feelings and sensations that life gives you.

Chapter 7

Turning in, turning on

How does the plumbing in your house work? When you run a bath or flush the toilet do you know where the water is actually coming from? Possibly not and yet you use these facilities and rely on them to be there, in working order, whenever you need them.

The same could be said of your body. It is there and working alright, so it is easy to assume it will be there and working alright all of the time — whether or not you understand how it functions. Amazingly, many people live their entire lives without that understanding. Many people enjoy excellent health without a clue about their body's physiology. Whether or not you are one of those people, learning more about how your body functions will definitely enhance your health. So, if you are eager to continue building upon the awareness and wellness you have gained since beginning your Movement Design practice, then look a little more closely at the workings of your body.

'Turning in' to focus on the physical components of movement will illuminate your understanding of your body's functions. Acquainting yourself with the practicalities of function will amplify your physical ease and control. Discovering your personal areas of limitation and excellence within your body's functions will create opportunities for pleasure, achievement and correction within your movement practice.

Over the following pages, the physical components of movement are illustrated through specific movements. There are six movements illustrated for each of six physical components. I suggest that you try all of the movements and then include in your regular practice the three or four that you find most challenging.

Posture movements

I would guess that your first reaction to the word 'posture' is to recall someone telling you to stand up straight in the manner of the military 'attention' stance. But posture is more than that — it is the springboard of movement; it is your position *during* as well as before and after movement.

Posture refers to the alignment of joints, the distribution of your weight, and the placement of your skeleton. Your posture is good or bad, but never non-existant and should, ideally, be a habitual carriage of your body that supports maximum health, safety and mobility. Should your postural habits be falling short of this ideal, then your best option is to retrain them into correctness, to re-habituate.

Correct posture creates health in your physical, mental and emotional natures. You see, because the skeleton lies embedded deep within your body, more than bone is affected by the quality of your posture. In particular, all muscle tissue and all major systems — such as nervous, digestive, circulatory — are made more healthy by the correctness of your posture. Your mood is also affected, as are your levels of vitality and alertness. Postural changes create fairly immediate alterations in your health and, to secure these benefits, repetition of the movements causing positive postural changes is advised. This is the re-habituation process: repetition of good postural habits in order to push the bad habits out of your postural repertoire.

When considering your posture, and when performing movements to correct or maintain it, always begin with your feet and move up your body. Try to retain a sense of lightness and length in your body and remember that support comes from above and attaches to the base of your sternum.

Posture movements

MOVEMENT 1:

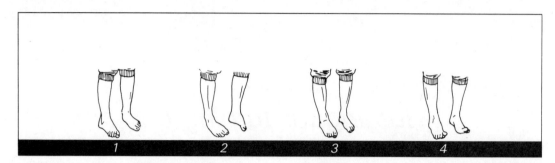

1 Stand or sit with your feet flat on the floor, hip-width apart. Keeping your feet pressed onto the floor, roll your ankles in towards each other.

2 Now roll them out, away from each other, as far as you can.

3 Roll your ankles back to centre and curl your toes under as tightly as you can. To extend this movement, you might try pulling your feet forwards by curling and uncurling your toes in this manner.

4 Now uncurl your toes and lift them as high as you can away from the floor. Be sure to keep the ball of your foot on the floor, though.

MOVEMENT 2:

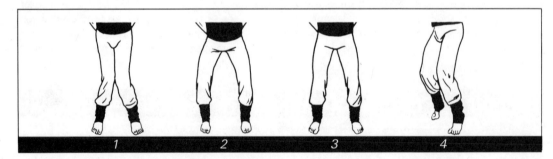

1 Stand or sit on the edge of a secure chair. Place your feet hip-width apart with the toes facing forwards. If you are standing, bend your knees but keep your heels flat on the floor. Relax your upper body. Now roll your knees in towards each other until they touch, or nearly so.

2 Now roll them out, away from each other as much as possible. Keep your feet as 'uninvolved' as you can.

3 Now place your knees so that they are in line with the centre of each foot. You may add a slight bouncing movement here to achieve a stronger sense of this position.

4 Keep your knees over the centre of your feet and then slowly 'peel' your heels off the floor so that you are balanced on the balls of your feet. Repeat this entire movement four times.

Posture movements

MOVEMENT 3:

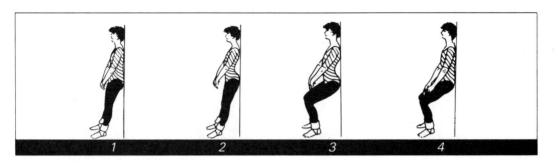

1 Lean against a wall with your feet shoulder-width apart, toes forwards and your heels 8-12 in (20-30cm) away from the wall. Keep your back straight and the back of your waist pressed firmly to the wall. Hold your chin comfortably close to your neck.

2 Arch your back so that only your tail-bone and the back of your shoulders are in contact with the wall.

3 Keep the arch as you bend your knees. This will cause you to slide down the wall a little distance. As you improve, you may wish to deepen the bend in your knees until you appear to be sitting on something invisible.

4 Keep your knees bent, however deeply you find comfortable, while you straighten your back once again. Remember to press your waist and middle back tightly to the wall. Now slide up the wall again into a standing position.

MOVEMENT 4:

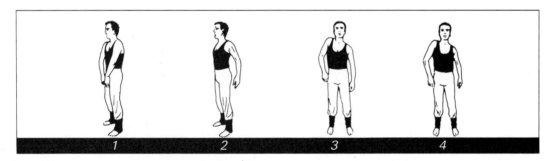

1 Stand or sit tall and think about your shoulders — both joints and muscles. As you breath out, wrap both shoulders forward as far as you can. Keep your arms just hanging, your neck relaxed and your chin level.

2 Now wrap your shoulders back as far as you can. Do not lift your shoulders at the same time, try to keep them level. Relax your neck.

3 Bring your shoulders out of the wrapping movement back to a central position. Now lift one shoulder as high as you can towards your ear. Press the other shoulder down as far as you can. Reverse this position.

4 Now combine these four positions into a rolling movement of the shoulders: lift, wrap forward, press down, wrap back, and lift again. You may do one shoulder at a time, or both together.

Posture movements

MOVEMENT 5:

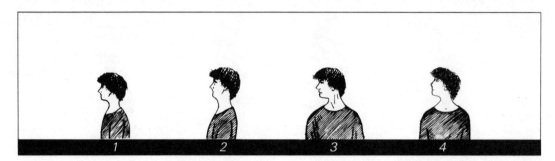

1 Stand or sit with your torso tall but relaxed. Rest your arms by your side. Bring your head forwards with a thrusting movement of the chin.

2 Now bring your head back as far as you can, as though tucking your chin in. This will show up a double-chin, even if you haven't got one!

3 Turn your head to one side as far as you can without turning your shoulder as well.

4 Now lift your chin 1-3 in (2-7 cm), keeping your head turned.

MOVEMENT 6:

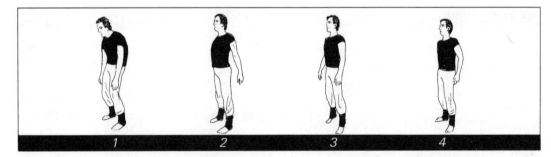

1 Stand how you like and then slump forwards to create the most slouchy body you can manage.

2 Reverse the slouch by arching your neck, shoulders and spine backwards. Your arms should hang slightly behind you, your chin should be lifted and your lower back may feel tight. Keep your legs very straight.

3 Relax your arms by your side and pull all of your parts back to their central position. Now push up onto the balls of your feet and pause there.

4 Keep all of the strength and balance that you used to stand on your toes while you lower your heels again. Breathe and repeat these positions.

Articulation movements

These occur at the point of movement itself — the joint. Articulation is the safe exploration of the range of movement available to you at each joint and includes the effect of movement on the fluids (lymph and synovia) and all the tissue surrounding each joint (tendon, ligament, muscle).

You may safely explore the range of movement available to you at any one joint by moving to the extremes of an articulation, making sure that you don't incur any degree of pain. So, for instance,

Movement 2 overleaf is a soothing articulation, but one that moves to the extremes of your mobility in the pelvic region. Combining articulations with the stretching that follows will increase your movement repertoire in general, and the ease with which you can articulate each joint in particular.

Articulation can have an 'unlocking' effect on your body — and the rest of your personality — which comes the closest to rejuvenation of any physical component of movement.

MOVEMENT 1:

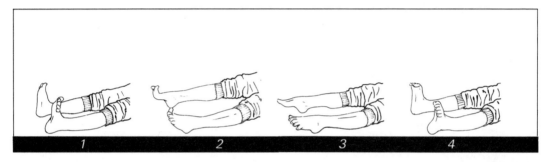

1 Sit comfortably or lie down. This movement may be performed with alternate feet or both feet simultaneously. Relax your toes as you flex your foot back towards your leg by reaching your heel away from you. You will feel a stretch in the muscles at the back of your leg.

2 Now reach the ball of your foot forwards, away from your leg. Do this while pulling the toes back towards your leg. (This gets easier with practice.)

3 Keep the ball of your foot reaching, but now stretch your toes forwards too. This stretch will tighten the arch in the sole of your foot.

4 Finally, curl your toes down as you flex your foot by reaching your heel away from your leg. Repeat these movements often.

Articulation movements

MOVEMENT 2:

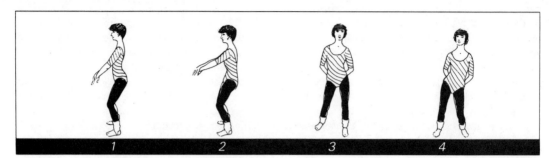

1 Stand with your feet at least hip-width apart, wider if you prefer. Let your arms hang loosely by your sides and bend both knees slightly. Keep your knees bent as you tilt your pelvis so that your tail-bone reaches out behind you. Do not arch the rest of your back — move just your pelvis.

2 Keep your knees bent and your arms hanging. Now tilt your pelvis so that your tail-bone is tucked under.

3 Still thinking of your pelvis, push one hip as far as you can to the side. Both knees are bent, although one more so than the other.

4 Reverse this movement by pushing the other hip to the side. Keep the rest of your body as relaxed as possible.

MOVEMENT 3:

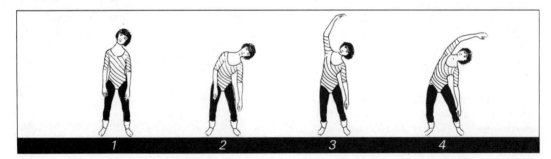

1 Stand with your feet shoulder-width apart and your toes pointing slightly out to each side. Bend both knees and keep them bent throughout. Let your arms hang at your sides and lower one ear towards the same shoulder.

2 As though someone were pulling you down by the ear, curve your torso more deeply to the side. Let your arms hang in front of you and keep your neck relaxed so that you aren't trying to hold your head up.

3 Hold this position (knees still bent) while you circle your upper arm out to your side and then up over your head. Breathe in as you raise your arm.

4 You may need to deepen the bend in your knees as you continue to circle your arm over your head and round down in front of you again. You can repeat this circling movement three or four times more, or you can lower your arm and uncurl your body from its lateral slumped position.

Articulation movements

MOVEMENT 4:

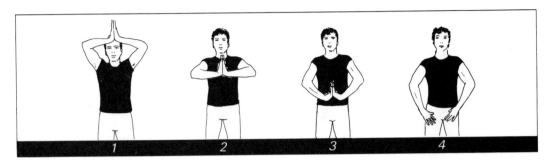

1 Stand or sit with your torso tall and straight. Press the palms of your hands together and hold them level with your forehead. Keep your shoulders relaxed and your elbows up and out to the side.

2 Increase the pressure between your palms as you lower your hands down to chest level, making sure you aren't tensing your neck.

3 Continue the downward movement of your hands. The pressure will remain but the 'heels' of your hands will pull away from one another. You will feel a considerable stretch in the palms of your hands and your fingers.

4 Continue the downward movement until your hands spring apart and the fingers spread as they are released from the pressure. Repeat.

MOVEMENT 5:

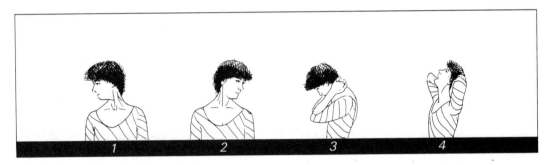

1 Stand or sit with your torso very tall and straight. Keep your shoulders level and free of tension. Now rest your chin forwards towards your neck and then roll your chin towards one shoulder. Your head will feel heavy.

2 Now roll your chin towards the other shoulder. Repeat this three or four times, all the while keeping your back tall and your shoulders relaxed.

3 Bring your chin back to centre but still dropped forwards. Bring your arms up and clasp both hands behind your neck. Hold this position for two breaths in and out. Let your arms feel heavy as well as your head.

4 Keep your hands clasped behind your neck but lift your chin towards the ceiling. Open your mouth as you do so. Give some of the weight of your head to the supporting arms. Repeat this whole movement.

Articulation movements

MOVEMENT 6:

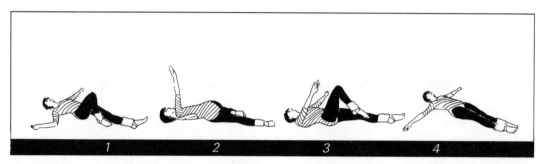

1 Lie flat on your back with one leg straight out along the floor, the other folded at the knee. Place the foot of your folded leg next to the knee of your straight leg. Stretch the arm opposite your folded leg straight out along the floor at shoulder-level. Let your other arm relax anywhere it wants.

2 Roll your folded leg across your straight leg until your knee nearly touches the floor. At the same time, bring your relaxed arm up in a straight line towards the ceiling and twist it. Twist all of the joints and feel all of the muscles stretch a little. Look towards this arm.

3 When you are ready, roll onto your back again. As you do so, lower the twisted arm down to your side. Keep it straight and twisted as it lowers.

4 Now stretch both legs straight along the floor and rest both arms straight by your sides. Breathe deeply and repeat on the other side.

Stretch movements

Stretch as a component of movement complements every articulation, and improves the ease with which a movement is performed. In addition, stretching has the effect of stimulating circulation, nerve response and respiratory function. It also greatly improves your mood and has a complementary effect on strength and posture.

Stretching is, in its ideal form, an uninhibited relaxation of the muscle tissue into its lengthened form. Gradual stretching increases the elasticity of the muscle tissue, thereby improving its responsiveness. Percussive or ballistic stretching (bouncing) should not be done as it may damage muscle tissue.

The best stretch-method is one that begins with the body in a safe, appropriate posture and enters into the stretch with adequate breath. The stretch may then be sustained, with breath, for a brief period before relaxing out of it. Alternatively, the stretch may be augmented at this point by relaxing and extending further into the stretch. You may require some practice before this feels comfortable to you. One way to make it comfortable is to use your own body-weight to extend the stretch for you. (For instance, Movement 7 in Chapter 3, Movements 3 and 4 below.) All that is needed is the correct posture, lots of breath, and a willingness to let your body, or part of your body, relax into feeling very heavy.

Stretch movements

MOVEMENT 1:

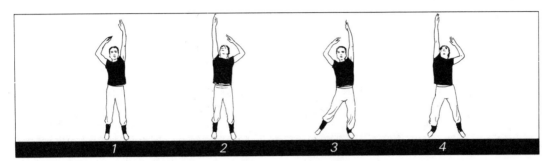

1 Stand with your feet hip-width apart, toes facing forwards. Raise both arms over your head. In this movement you may either look forwards or up towards your hands. Stretch one arm up as far as you can as you let the other relax at the elbow.

2 Now stretch your other arm and let your first arm relax.

3 Extend this movement by spreading your feet shoulder-width apart. This time, as you stretch one arm, bend the corresponding knee. You will feel this stretch along the length of your torso and more deeply into your waist.

4 Now stretch your other arm and bend your other knee.

MOVEMENT 2:

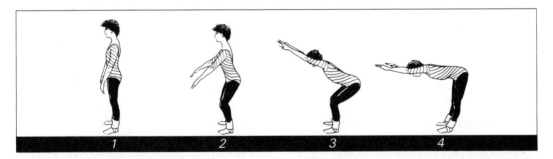

1 Stand with your feet comfortably apart, toes forwards. Let your arms rest by your side.

2 Stretch your arms straight in front of you at shoulder-level. At the same time, bend your knees and reach your tail-bone back. Leave your heels on the floor.

3 Keep about the same degree of bend in your knees. Continue to reach your tail-bone back and your arms forwards until you feel that your body is a straight line from tail-bone to fingertips. Let your head rest between your arms and look towards the floor.

4 Now stretch your legs to eliminate much or all of the bend. Hold this position for two or three breaths then bend your knees and come to a standing position once again.

Stretch movements

MOVEMENT 3:

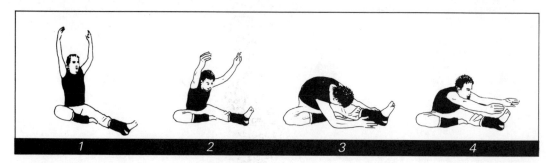

1 Sit tall with one leg stretched straight along the floor, your other leg folded at the knee. Let your folded knee rest sideways towards the floor, supported with a cushion if you like. Raise both arms up over your head and look forwards.

2 Now lean forwards from your hips, keeping your back as straight as you can. Try not to hold your breath.

3 When you have leaned as far as you want to, lower your arms to the floor beside your lower leg and drop your forehead towards your knee.

4 Now stretch your arms towards your feet and look towards your toes. At the same time, press your chest near to your thigh. Breathe deeply.

MOVEMENT 4:

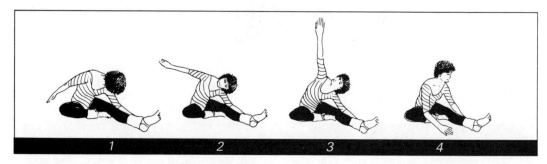

1 Sit curled forwards with one leg straight and the other folded at the knee. Put some of your upper body-weight onto one arm and stretch your other arm back by your side.

2 Continue to stretch this arm and, as you breathe in, circle it back and up over your head. Keep your torso as near to your leg as possible. Your straight leg may wish to bend slightly: let it.

3 Circle your arm right up over your head and then look at your hand. Breathe out as you complete the circle forward. Now repeat with other arm.

4 Place both hands flat on the floor beside your leg and use their strength to lift your upper body into a tall sitting position.

Note: Movements 3 and 4 may be performed in sequence.

Stretch movements

MOVEMENT 5:

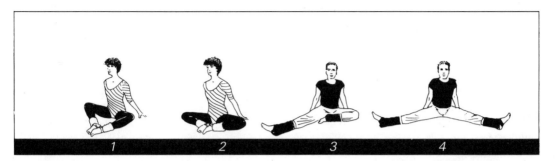

1 Sit tall with the soles of your feet pressed together a comfortable distance from you. Let your knees relax open towards the floor. Place your hands behind your hips for support.

2 Bring your feet as close to your body as you can. This will increase the sense of stretch in your inner thigh muscles. Either hold on to your ankles or place your hands behind your hips for support.

3 Sit tall with one leg stretched along the floor as far to the side as you find comfortable. Fold your other leg at the knee and bring the heel close to your torso. Place your hands behind your hips for support.

4 Sit tall with both legs stretched straight along the floor as far apart as you find comfortable. Give support by placing your hands behind your hips. Wiggle your toes and roll your legs gently in and out, once or twice.

Note: You may select one of these stretches if you prefer, or perform all four in a slow, gradual sequence.

MOVEMENT 6:

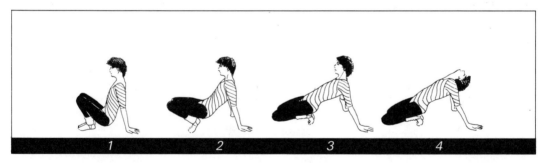

1 Sit with your feet tucked close to your hips and your hands shoulder-width apart close to your back. Now lift your tail-bone off the floor and rock it gently back and forth towards your heels.

2 Press onto the balls of your feet. Your knees will move forwards and you will begin to feel a stretch in your arms and shoulders.

3 Push your knees as far forwards as you comfortably can. Keep your head lifted to look along the front of your body. This is a powerful stretch. You may hold this position or come quickly out of it.

4 This part is entirely optional. In the fullness of the stretch, lower your head gently behind you. Hold it for one breath and then lift it again.

Strength movements

Strength is the opposite of stretch in that the muscle tissue is in its shortened form. The term most often used is 'contracted'. A contracted muscle generally becomes a prominant one while it remains contracted (a stretched muscle tends to flatten), but building strength does not necessarily leave you with permanently bulgy muscles — you'll have to try a different method from this one to end up with those. The strength you will acquire through your Movement Design practice is a subtle, supportive strength that enhances all of your movements and brings gracefulness to them.

Strength may be gained by opposing your position, or the direction of your movement, with weight or tension. Just about every movement or position you ever do needs strength, because strength doesn't apply only to those muscles that you find most obvious, it also applies to deep muscle and to the hidden strengths required of your internal organs.

It is important to maintain correct posture throughout these movements. Only then can you be certain that your strength and posture support one another in their improvements. Strength capabilities are enhanced by stretching and appropriate breathing patterns — those that leave you with sufficient oxygen in your system to complete your strength movement without cramping or pain.

MOVEMENT 1:

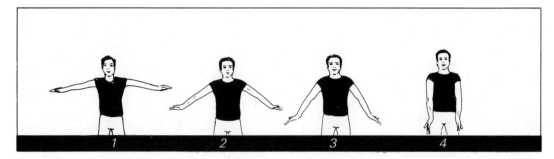

1 Stand or sit with your arms stretched straight out to your sides at shoulder-level. Keep the sense of stretch while you twist every part of your arm.

2 Keep the twist and the stretch while you pulse both arms back and down in small stages. From the shoulders, pulse to chest level.

3 Pulse back and down to waist area. Keep your arms straight and keep breathing.

4 Pulse back and down to the hips. Now reverse the movement by twisting your arms in the opposite direction and pulsing your arms upwards. Do not allow yourself to become breathless in this movement.

Strength movements

MOVEMENT 2:

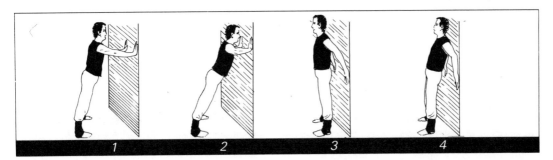

1 Stand facing a wall with your body upright. Place your hands at shoulder-level flat against the wall and straighten your arms. Spread your feet shoulder-width apart and move them back so that they are about 8 in (20cm) behind the line of your shoulders. You should feel your arms working to support your body-weight.

2 Keep your heels flat on the floor and bend your elbows. Your head and chest will move closer to the wall causing your arms to work even harder. In this movement, your ankles are the point of pivot: do not bend at the hips or waist. Repeat these two movements up to 12 times. Breathe freely.

3 Now turn your back to the wall and place your hands flat against the wall shoulder-width apart at hip-level. Straighten your arms. As in the previous version, move your feet away from the wall about 8 in (20cm). Your legs and body are in a straight line.

4 Now bend your elbows so that your body moves back towards the wall. Keep your body straight, the point of pivot is the ankles. You may make this movement as large or as small as you like. Adjust the distance of your feet from the wall to make this easier or more difficult. Repeat these movements up to 12 times.

MOVEMENT 3:

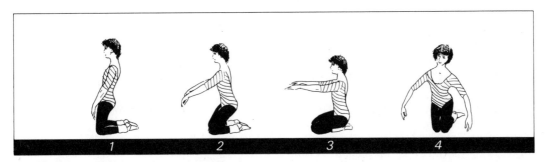

1 Kneel tall with your knees and lower legs at least hip-width apart. Let your arms rest comfortably by your sides. Keeping your middle body straight, move back and forth, pivoting from your knees. You will feel the effort in your thigh muscles.

2 Return to an upright position and then bend at the hips and lower your hips towards your heels. Stop well before you rest onto your heels and then lift your hips again.

3 Again, lower your hips but this time do sit on your heels. Rest there if you like, then lift your hips once again, keeping your back straight.

4 From the tall position, lower your hips towards one heel. Lift your hips again and lower them towards your other heel. Your middle body will curve.

Strength movements

MOVEMENT 4:

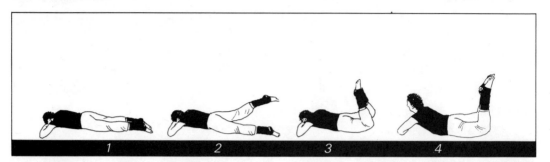

1 Stretch out on the floor, lying on your abdomen. Place your hands — palms down — under your forehead, elbows out to the sides.

2 Now stretch one leg and raise it a small distance off the floor. This movement is from the hip so your leg remains stretched. Do not lift your hip, keep the front of your pelvis pressed firmly to the floor. Then lower your leg and reverse.

3 Stretch both your legs and fold them back at the knees, letting your ankles cross if they want to. Now raise your knees a small distance off the floor.

4 Rest a moment then raise your knees again. This time, lift your head and shoulders out of their resting position and look forwards. Repeat.

MOVEMENT 5:

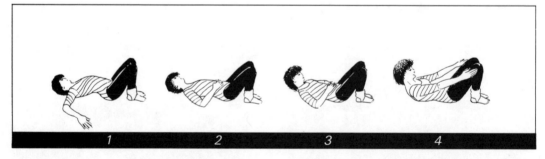

1 Lie flat on your back on the floor, bring your knees up and place your feet flat on the floor. Keep your feet and knees hip-width apart. Relax your arms and shoulders and bring your chin comfortably close to your neck. Now tilt your pelvis to create an arch behind your waist. You will feel your tail-bone pressing down towards the floor.

2 Now tilt your pelvis in the opposite direction so that you feel the back of your waist pressing firmly onto the floor. Hold it there. Cross your hands over your navel.

3 Keep the back of your waist on the floor while you tuck your chin to your neck. Now lift your head and shoulders. Look towards your knees.

4 Hold this position but stretch your arms towards your knees. Do not try to sit up straight. Hold for one breath in and out then rest back on the floor again.

Strength movements

MOVEMENT 6:

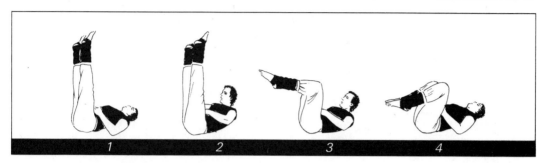

1 Lie flat with the back of your waist pressing onto the floor. Cross your hands over your navel. Stretch both legs up towards the ceiling and keep your feet relaxed. Do not worry if you cannot straighten your legs.

2 Keep your legs stretching while you curl your head and shoulders up.

3 Hold the curl, take a breath, and then fold your legs so your thighs are vertical and your lower legs are at right angles to them. Keep your feet relaxed.

4 Now lower your head and shoulders and bring your knees close to your torso, all at once. Relax completely and repeat.

Balance movements

Balance is the art of stillness, however brief or prolonged. You may think of balance, too, as an awareness of opposition: for every forward there is a backward, for every extension there is a contraction, for every stillness there is a backdrop of movement. A sense of correctness accompanies a balance, an ease and something very like contentment. For these reasons, balance may become a very energizing part of your movement practice — especially when you realize that you don't have to perform arabesques to achieve it. Posture, articulation, stretch and strength, are all used within a balance and the pleasure of balance is increased if your breathing is made to help you. This can be achieved by taking long, deep breaths once the point of balance is reached.

MOVEMENT 1:

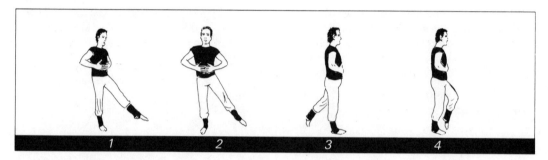

1 Stand tall with your hands holding the sides of your ribs. Stretch one leg forwards, toes pointing, and raise your leg off the floor.

2 Keeping your toes raised just off the floor, circle your leg around to the side. Keep your body as still and upright as you can.

3 Now circle your leg behind you. Keep your pelvis upright so that you don't lean forward.

4 Now bend your knee and bring your leg under and forwards again. This time step on to it and repeat the movement using your other leg.

Balance movements

MOVEMENT 2:

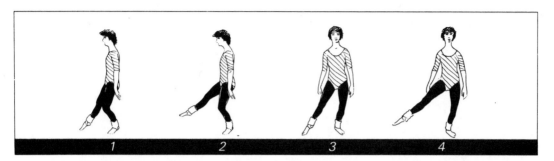

1 Stand tall with your feet hip-width apart and your arms by your sides. Now bend one leg and let the other slide forwards, stretching your toes. Let your arms move slightly behind you to help you balance. Look forwards.

2 Hold your front leg straight and raise it, from the hip, in front of you. Keep your supporting leg bent at the knee. Lower your leg and repeat this on the other side.

3 Stand tall with your feet shoulder-width apart, the toes facing slightly out to the sides. Now bend one leg and let your other one slide sideways with the toes stretched. Raise your arms a little to help balance.

4 Keep your leg stretching to the side as you raise it off the floor. Your supporting leg remains bent at the knee. Lower your leg and repeat on the other side.

MOVEMENT 3:

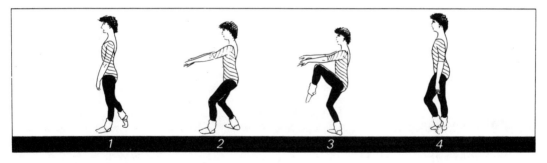

1 Stand tall with your arms by your sides. Now reach one leg straight behind you and transfer half your body-weight onto it.

2 Putting your weight evenly between your two legs, lower your hips as though you are about to sit on a stool. Raise your arms in front of you to help you balance. 'Sit' as low as you can, keeping your heels flat on the floor.

3 Hold this balance, then slowly raise your front knee up towards the ceiling. Keep the other leg bent and your torso straight.

4 Lower your lifted leg onto the floor so that your feet are side by side. Immediately stand and relax. Repeat on the other side.

Balance movements

MOVEMENT 4:

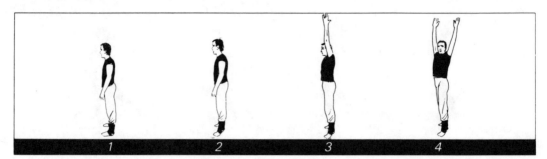

1 Stand tall with your arms by your sides and your weight over the balls of your feet. Look forwards (it helps to find a specific point to look at).

2 Raise yourself onto the balls of your feet. Keep your arms hanging loosely by your sides.

3 Hold your heels off the floor and slowly stretch both arms over your head. Keeping your torso tall will help you to balance. Look forwards.

4 Keep your heels lifted and your arms stretched. Now slowly twist your torso so that you are looking to one side. Turn back to centre and reverse the twist. Lower your heels and your arms, then repeat the whole sequence.

MOVEMENT 5:

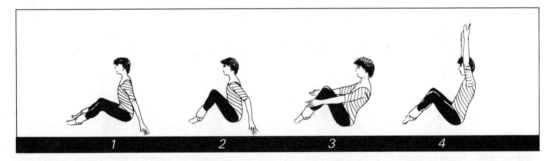

1 Sit tall with your knees lifted slightly in front of you. Keep your feet stretched on the floor about shoulder-width apart. Rest your arms by your sides.

2 Keep the height in your torso as you bring your knees a little closer to your torso. Keep your feet stretching and your toes tightly pressed onto the floor.

3 Use your toes to push yourself back to a balance on your tail-bone. You may wish to lift your arms slightly to help you balance. Keep your back very straight. Look forwards.

4 Hold this balance while you stretch both arms up over your head. Try to hold them in a straight line with your torso. Breathe, then rest and repeat.

Balance movements

MOVEMENT 6:

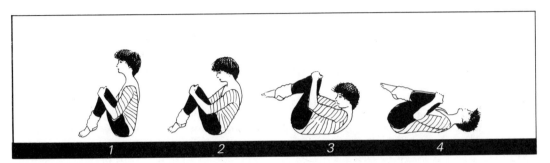

1 Sit very tall while you hug your knees as close to your chest as you can. Look forwards.

2 Now round your lower back. Keep hold of your knees even though they will move a little distance forwards to help you balance.

3 Continue to round your back so that you roll slowly backwards along your spine. Keep hold of your knees and use their distance from your chest to help you balance. Look forwards and try not to wobble from side to side.

4 Finally, rest down flat on your back and keep hugging your knees.

Breath movements

This really is a component of movement. It is, in fact, the most constant movement/stillness pattern you experience.

Adequate and appropriate breathing patterns are essential for healthy body functioning, especially if your body is working to improve strength, stretch and movement capabilities. Adequacy in breath implies a sufficiency of oxygen inhaled to supply your body's needs and a thorough exhalation, when some waste products are flushed from your system. Inadequacy in breath results in cramp, tension, pain, and impairment of muscular function.

Breath can relax you — especially the breath out — as well as help you to concentrate. It is useful to become aware of your manner of breathing in a variety of situations and during various movements. Once noted, you may alter your breathing patterns to make them appropriate to the movements you are doing. So, for instance, a recommendation to breathe out at one point may enable you to fulfil a movement or become more aware of a stretch or articulation. Breathing in at another point in your movement may give nourishment to the movement at the point when your body is most under stress.

MOVEMENT 1:

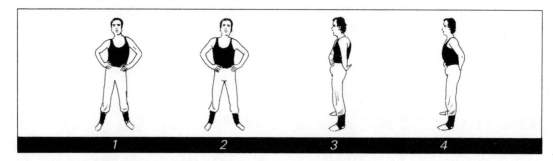

1 Stand or sit tall and place your hands on your hips. Keep your shoulders relaxed and think only of your lungs and rib cage. Now shift your ribs to one side.

2 Now to the other side. Keep your pelvis still and your neck relaxed.

3 Imagine your ribs lifting slightly and now shift your rib cage backwards. This is a small movement, so keep the rest of your body relaxed.

4 Now move your rib cage forwards. This is easier. Repeat the entire movement.

Breath movements

MOVEMENT 2:

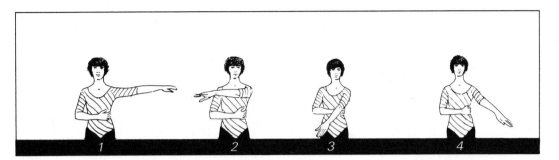

1 Stand or sit with one arm stretched to your side at shoulder-level. The other arm is crossed in front with the hand gripping the side of your ribs.

2 Begin to circle your straight arm around in front of you at shoulder-level.

3 When you can circle it no further, begin to lower it in front of you.

4 Keep your arm straight and swing it down and across your body. Return it to the starting position and repeat on this side, then reverse and repeat.

MOVEMENT 3:

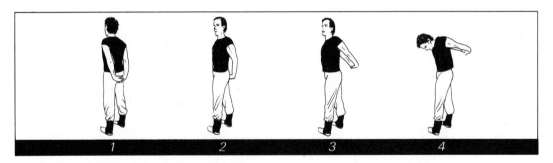

1 Stand or sit tall on the edge of your chair. Clasp your hands behind you level with your tail-bone. Take a good breath in.

2 Keep your hands clasped as you twist your torso to one side. Breathe out as you twist.

3 Maintain the twist and raise your clasped hands up behind you as you take a good breath in.

4 Keep your hands clasped and lifted, keep your torso twisted. Now breathe out and slump your head, shoulders and chest slightly forwards. Return to the central, untwisted position and reverse this movement.

Breath movements

MOVEMENT 4:

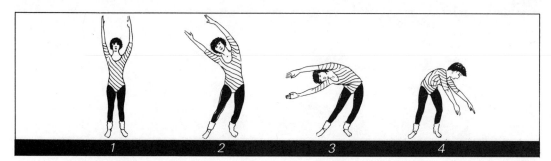

1 Stand tall with your feet shoulder-width apart and your toes facing slightly out to the sides. Raise your arms above your head and breathe in.

2 Keep your arms straight as you swing them both down and to one side. At the same time, bend the knee that is opposite the direction of your arms so that your weight moves onto that leg.

3 Continue the downward swing of your arms. Your torso will curl and the bend in your knee will deepen. Breathe out all the while.

4 Your arms will swing into a position parallel with your legs and then, beyond that position, to your other side. Once there, begin to retrace the path your arms took in their swing down. Breathe in as you lift them into the starting position. Now reverse this movement as you breathe out.

MOVEMENT 5:

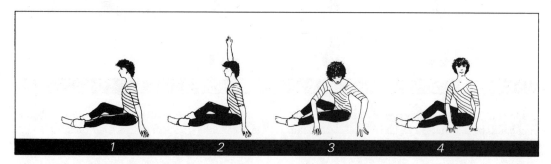

1 Sit on the floor with one leg stretched straight out in front of you, your other knee lifted slightly. Rest your fingertips on the floor beside your hips.

2 Breathe in as you raise one arm up over your head.

3 Breathe out as you lower this arm across your body to place your fingertips beside your other hand. Now your torso is both curled and twisted. Look at your hands. You may hold this position for two or three breaths if you like.

4 Breathe in as you lengthen your torso out of the curl, but maintain the twist. Then bring your torso back to the starting position as you breathe out. Repeat this movement on the other side. Repeat twice more with your other knee lifted.

Breath movements

MOVEMENT 6:

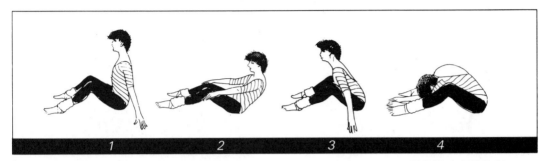

1 Sit on the floor with your torso lengthened, your legs slightly folded and your feet shoulder-width apart. Stretch your toes and breathe in.

2 As you breathe out, round your back and let it slump behind you. Let your head rest forwards. Try to keep your arms relaxed near to, but not gripping, your thighs.

3 Breathe in again as you lengthen your spine and lean it forwards — all at once. Keep your knees lifted and your arms relaxed. The leaning movement is from your hips, your back should be as straight as you can manage.

4 Breathe out as you round your back forwards. Rest here for three or four breaths allowing your upper body, your arms, shoulders and head to feel heavy. Then uncurl and repeat the entire movement.

Chapter 8
You did it . . . now do it again!

Congratulations, you have come a long way. The reward belongs to no one else because the changes you have brought about, however small they may seem, bring with them an increase in awareness, an increase in balance, an improvement in your health. You have taken the brave step of observing, acknowledging and allowing your own unique blend of body, mind and emotion. You have designed your movements to be more appropriate to your personality and your life. You have made progress.

Now that you know how it's done, you can do it again. You have all that is necessary to do so contained within you. You have experienced the Movement Design process and achieved some of the benefits

that result. Now you need only continue your practice in order to keep progress as a constant presence in your life.

Before you begin your second round of progress, however, consider one more application of the Movement Design process. This application deals with those times of discomfort or illness that everyone confronts at times. These may be occasions when you feel that movement causes problems or discomfort, or when it feels like the very last thing you want to do. The following examples may provide you with the movement answers to these situations.

Try them now if you wish, so that you know they are there when you need them — they work wonders.

Task-related movements

Apart from standard postural changes, which you have already worked with, there are some corrections or alterations you may make to the movements and positions you perform during the course of any one day. These changes will benefit your health, vitality and alertness while performing task movements.

MOVEMENT 1:
For reaching something at a low level or moving onto the floor.

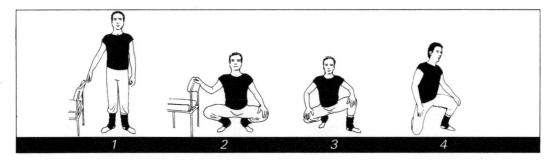

1 Stand and hold on to a worktop, chair or wall. Keep your heels apart and your torso straight. Do not curve your back. Keep looking forwards.

2 Push your tail-bone down towards the floor in a straight line keeping your back straight. Your heels will lift and your knees should move out to the sides.

3 Now swing your tail-bone over one heel. Push your other foot further to your side and lower your heel. You may reverse this position at any time.

4 Lower your other knee (the tightly folded one) onto the floor so that your weight is shared between the flat foot and this knee.

Task-related movements

MOVEMENT 2:

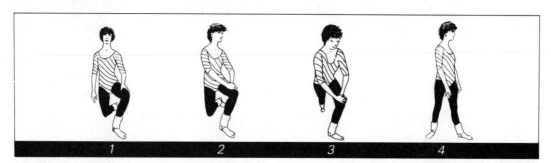

1 Kneel tall on one knee only. Pull your other knee up to one side at hip-level so that your foot is flat. (This is a very secure and open position.)

2 Now turn your torso to face your lifted knee. At the same time, curl your back set of toes under.

3 Use the back set of toes to push you up and forwards along the line of your lifted knee and thigh. Use the strength in your thighs to lift your body-weight — do *not* use the strength in your back.

4 Keep your momentum forwards until you are able to bring your back leg forwards in a step.

MOVEMENT 3:

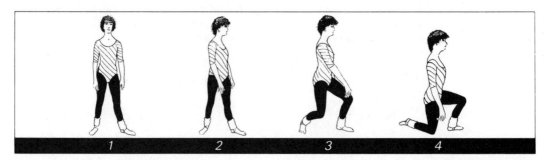

1 Stand tall with your feet shoulder-width apart. Leave one set of toes facing forwards, turn the others out to one side.

2 Twist your torso to face the same direction as the turned-out toes.

3 Slowly bend your other leg as you move your weight onto the turned-out leg. Keep lowering your folded knee towards the floor as you turn.

4 Finally, rest your folded knee on the floor. You should be in a tall kneeling position facing the turned-out toes.

Task-related movements

MOVEMENT 4:
To roll in and out of bed while pregnant or if suffering from a bad back.

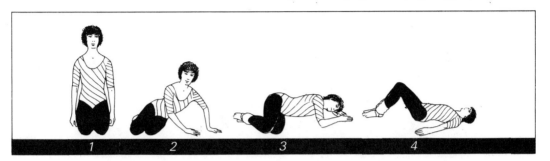

1 Sit on the edge of your bed, or sit on your heels on the floor.

2 Place both hands on the bed or floor, to one side of your pelvis. Use the strength in your arms to lower yourself onto your side by 'walking' your hands away from you.

3 When you are resting on your side, have a moments pause with your knees and your arms folded. Imagine tension draining from your body.

4 Give a final push with your arms and roll onto your back.

MOVEMENT 5:
If you spend all day on your feet, this will help prevent varicose vein problems, backache and arthritic pains.

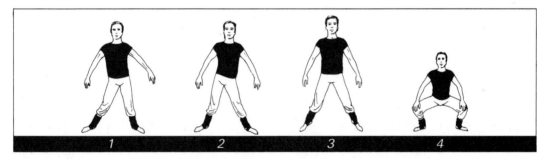

1 Stand tall with your feet just wider than shoulder-width apart. Turn your toes to face out to the sides. Let your arms relax by your sides. Keeping your legs straight, push your legs and hips to one side.

2 Then the other. You will feel this in the top, inner thighs as well as the hip joints.

3 Bring your pelvis back to centre and lift both heels. Keep your legs straight and balance for a few seconds.

4 Lower your heels again and at the same time bend your knees so that they open out slightly to the sides. Repeat this entire movement.

Task-related movements

MOVEMENT 6:

These will help you to save your back and general posture from long-term or chronic ailments.

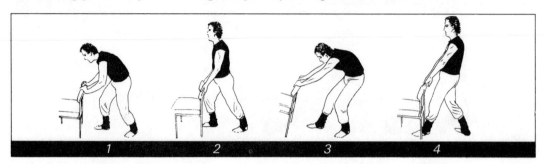

1 A common, but incorrect, stance while pushing, often resulting from the handles of a trolley or pram being at the wrong height.

2 Instead walk 'into' the object being pushed so that your body is a straight line from heel to head. Keep your chin lifted and your elbows back as you push. You want your arms and legs to do the hard work, not your back and neck.

3 A common, but incorrect, stance while pulling, which may be due to weak arms or abdomen.

4 Instead straighten your back and use your body-weight and the strength in your arms to exert the pulling force.

MOVEMENT 7:

Gardening, bathing the kids, or other awkward-height activities are made less uncomfortable by using this movement as an interlude.

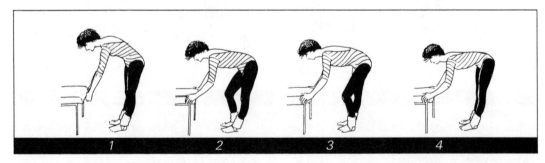

1 A common stance while bending over. This is often unavoidable due to the design or height of the object being worked with (for instance, a bathtub). However, the lower back is in danger and tension and fatigue will mount in the legs, shoulders and neck.

2 For relief, rest your hands or elbows against the edge of the object. Now straighten your back. Bend one knee leaving that heel on the floor, keeping your other leg straight. Keep your head lowered to relax your neck muscles. Your breathing should be steady.

3 Now bend the other knee and straighten the first leg. This movement will mobilize the pelvis and soothe your lower back.

4 Now straighten both legs. Keep your back straight and bend your arms just slightly. The result is a gentle stretch to the lower back muscles.

Task-related movements

MOVEMENT 8:

Sedentary job? This will save your back, hips and swollen ankles — and it's alright to do in public!

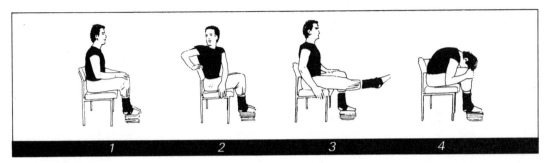

1 Sit tall and place your feet on an object about 6 in (15cm) high.

2 Now twist your torso and bring one arm behind you, the other across your body. Hold onto the back and side of your chair while you breathe deeply in and out. Repeat this twist on your other side.

3 Turn back to centre and stretch one leg up in front of you. You do not have to straighten it. Keep your back tall while you point and flex this foot. Now rotate your foot in both directions. Repeat with your other leg.

4 Place both feet back on their support again. Sit tall with your arms relaxed. Now breathe out and let your waist drop back, your head and shoulders drop forwards. Rest here for three or four breaths.

Movements to relieve ailments

You may obtain temporary relief from some chronic ailments by using movement to minimize their discomfort. In some cases movement may even begin to remedy the problem at its source. Do not be wary of using movement in this way — movement generally stimulates your body's self-healing capabilities so that you will recover more quickly. Your body will respond well to movement during these times.

MOVEMENT 1:
For relief of headaches — three versions.

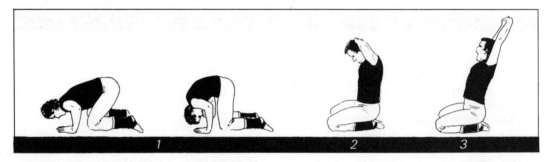

1 Go down onto your hands and knees. Be sure that your knees and hands are shoulder-width apart. Now lower your forehead down onto the floor.

Supporting your body-weight in your hands and arms, roll forwards onto the top of your head. Hold this position for about 30 seconds then roll onto your forehead and repeat it after a pause. Keep your breathing relaxed.

2 Sit on your heels with your back straight and your hands clasped behind your head. Now lower your head forwards, keeping the rest of your back upright. Let your jaw hang slack. Hold this position for 30 seconds.

3 Sitting on your heels with your back straight, raise both arms up over your head. Lock your fingers together and gently pulse your arms backwards from the shoulders. Keep your neck relaxed and your jaw slack.

Movements to relieve ailments

MOVEMENT 2:
To ease chronic headache or pain and stiffness in the neck, shoulder or upper spine.

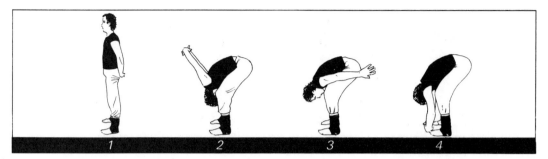

1 Stand tall with your feet hip-width apart and your hands clasped behind you level with your tail-bone. Feel your shoulder blades pinch together. Look forwards.

2 Curl forwards towards the floor (see Movement 7, page 36) letting your clasped arms circle above your head as you do so. Keep your hands clasped and hold the full position for at least one breath in and out.

3 Maintain the curl of your body but lower your hands down towards your tail-bone. Unclasp your hands and allow your arms to slide down the side of your legs to the floor.

4 Give your head and arms a gentle shake to help release tension. Then uncurl *slowly* from this position keeping your knees bent and your head hanging until the last moment. Stand and repeat this when you are ready.

MOVEMENT 3
To relieve the discomfort of menstrual pains and/or constipation.

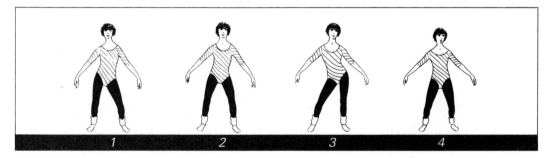

1 Stand tall or lean slightly forwards using the back of a chair as a support. Place your feet at least shoulder-width apart and bend both knees. Keep your knees bent as you begin to circle your pelvis, moving first to one side.

2 Then tilt your pelvis back. Your ribs should remain still and central.

3 Continue to circle your pelvis around but this time towards your other side. Relax your breathing.

4 Now tilt your pelvis forwards as you complete the circle. This movement may be done fast or slow. Try circling in both directions. Finish by straightening your legs and coming into a normal standing position.

Movements to relieve ailments

MOVEMENT 4:

To improve the circulation to the legs and feet: for cold, swollen, tired legs or varicose veins.

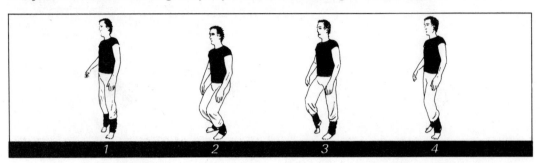

1 Stand tall with your feet hip-width apart. Now lift and lower your heels several times. Keep your ankles upright as you do this: do not allow them to buckle out to the sides. Relax your arms by your sides.

2 When you have done the first part several times, have a rest by lowering your heels and bouncing your knees forwards several times. This will give instant relief from any tension created by the heel-lift.

3 Stand straight again. Lift one heel and push the knee of this leg forwards. Keep your other leg straight and your upper body still and tall.

4 Now lower your heel and straighten the leg. Lift your other heel and push that knee forwards. This is a 'cycling' movement. Repeat.

MOVEMENT 5:

To relieve varicose veins or very tired, swollen legs and feet.

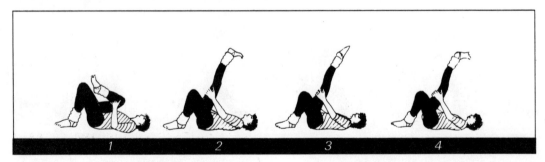

1 Lie flat on your back with both knees lifted and both feet flat on the floor. Now lift one knee towards the ceiling and use both hands to hold onto your thigh.

2 Stretch your lower leg up towards the ceiling also. You do not need to straighten your leg, just stretch it. Keep hold of your thigh.

3 In this position, point and flex your foot several times. Keep your chin close to your neck and remember to breathe.

4 Also in this position, rotate your foot from the ankle. Then bend your knee, place your foot back onto the floor and reverse this movement.

Movements to relieve ailments

MOVEMENT 6:
To ease the discomfort of a bad back or a feeling of congestion in the pelvic region.

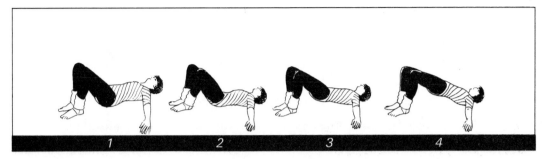

1 Lie flat on your back with your knees lifted and your feet on the floor about hip-width apart. Press the back of your waist firmly onto the floor. Rest your arms a little distance from your sides.

2 Think of your spine and slowly raise your tail-bone towards the ceiling, keeping the back of your waist pressed onto the floor at this point.

3 Now lift your pelvis and waist away from the floor. Keep your rib cage pressed onto the floor as much as you can.

4 Now lift your rib cage off the floor so that you have created a straight line — along the back of your body — between knees and shoulders. Hold this position for a few seconds and then reverse it, slowly lowering back into the resting position. Repeat this movement several times quite slowly.

MOVEMENT 7:
To relieve acute backache.

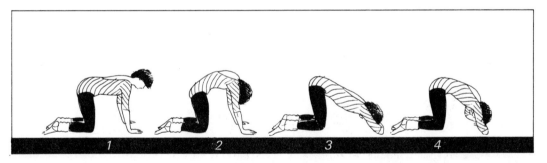

1 Move onto your hands and knees with both hands and knees shoulder-width apart. Lower your head to relax your neck muscles.

2 Now tilt your pelvis so that your tail-bone tucks forwards and under. This will cause your lower and middle back to lift or round in an arch. Relax this arch then repeat slowly several times. Breathe deeply.

3 Now lower onto your elbows so that your tail-bone faces the ceiling and your back is a fairly straight line down to your neck. You may find this a restful position in itself. Keep your head lowered forwards.

4 Tilt your pelvis to bring your tail-bone down and forwards. This is a small movement. Your lower back will round slightly. Repeat. Breathe deeply.

Movements to relieve ailments

MOVEMENT 8:

To relieve backache and maintain mobility in the back for those whose discomfort is not severe.

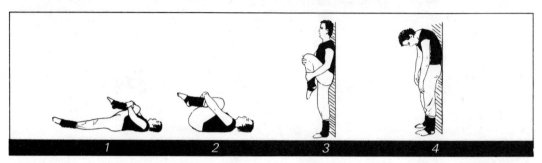

1 Lie flat on your back with one leg stretched out along the floor (either straight or slightly bent). Fold your other leg and hug that knee close to your chest. The back of your waist will press onto the floor. Be certain to keep your chin close to your neck. Hold this position for two or three breaths. Now try it with your other leg if you can.

2 Bring both knees close to your chest and hug them there for one minute.

3 Stand with your back tightly pressed against a wall. Lift one knee up and hug it close to your chest. Keep as much of your spine in contact with the wall as you can manage. Hold this for three or four breaths. Reverse if you can.

4 Place both feet on the floor and press the back of your waist and your middle back against the wall. Now slump your head, shoulders and arms forwards. Just relax as best you can for at least one breath.

Movements for special circumstances

There are always movements that are able to provide support for your entire personality during times of special need. These occasions are often those in which you may feel 'frozen' and incapable of movement, such as in times of grief or trauma. It is precisely these times, and times of great physical change, that benefit profoundly from movement. Remember, the most constant goal within your movement practice is that of progress and wellness. Therefore, it is essential that movement is not left out of your life at times when you, perhaps, feel less inclined to do it.

Pregnancy
Three new movements, plus a selection from those you have already performed.

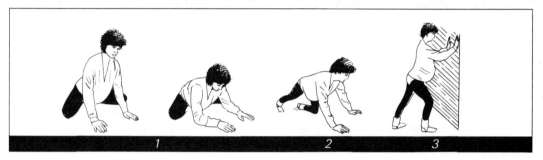

1 Sit on your heels with your knees well apart. Lean forwards onto your hands, keeping your arms straight. You may rock backwards and forwards in this position if you like. Keep your torso straight and lengthened.

Keep your tail-bone over your heels but now rest down onto your elbows. You may keep your head lifted — for instance, while reading — or you may rest it forwards to relax your neck and facial muscles. You may rock backwards and forwards in this position too.

2 From a hands-and-knees position, stretch one leg behind you and curl that set of toes under. Now move that same heel back to feel a stretch in your calf muscle. Move the heel forwards to relax the stretch. Repeat this often and then try it on the other leg.

3 Stand facing a wall with your hands at shoulder level against it. Stretch one leg back and bend your front leg. Now check that both heels are flat on the floor and both sets of toes face forwards. Hold this position while you move your front knee to and from the wall. Keep your body straight (don't let your tail-bone stick out) and you will feel this in your calf muscle. Repeat this movement on your other side.

TRY THESE TOO:

Movements 2 and 3 from The basic 12 (pages 33 and 34)

Movements 10 and 11 from The top 20 (pages 58 and 59)

Movements 1, 3 and 4 from the Posture movements section (pages 72 and 73)

Movements 1, 2, 4, 5 and 6 from the Articulation movements section (pages 75, 76, 77 and 78)

Movements 5 and 6 from the Stretch movements section (page 81)

Movement 3 from the Breath movements section (page 91)

Movements 1, 2, 3, 4, 6 and 7 from the Task-related movements section (pages 95, 96, 97 and 98)

Movements 3, 4, 5, 6 and 7 from the Movements to relieve ailments section (pages 101, 102 and 103)

The sleeping twist (page 108)

Movements for special circumstances

Post-natal recovery

One new movement, plus a selection from those you have already performed.

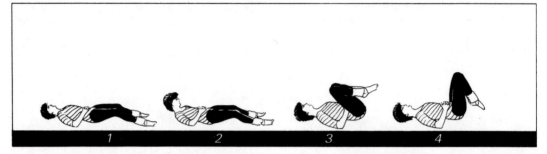

1 Lie flat on the floor with your knees slightly lifted. Keep your feet and knees hip-width apart and cross your hands over your navel. Now press the back of your waist onto the floor.

2 Tuck your chin in towards your neck and lift your head and shoulders. Look towards your knees. Do *not* try to sit up. Hold for 5 seconds then relax back.

3 Lie flat again but this time lift first one knee, then the other, up towards your chest. Keep your lower legs relaxed and your hands on your navel.

4 Now move your knees forwards, away from your chest, until they are vertical, at right angles to the floor. Keep your lower legs relaxed and the back of your waist touching the floor. Bring your knees to your chest again and repeat slowly.

TRY THESE TOO:

Movements 2, 3 and 7 from The basic 12 (pages 33, 34 and 36)

Movements 9, 11 and 12 from The top 20 (pages 57, 59 and 60)

Movements 2, 3 and 4 from the Posture movements section (pages 72 and 73)

Movements 1, 2, 3 and 6 from the Articulation movements section (pages 75, 76 and 78)

Movements 1, 4, 5 and 6 from the Stretch movements section (pages 79, 80 and 81)

Movements 1, 2, 3, 4 (steps 1 and 2) and 5 from the Strength movements section (pages 82, 83 and 84)

Movement 6 from the Breath movements section (page 93)

Movements 1, 2, 3, 5, 6 and 7 from the Task-related movements section (pages 95, 96, 97 and 98)

Movements 1, 3, 4 and 7 from the Movements to relieve ailments section (pages 100, 101, 102 and 103)

Movements for special circumstances

Illness and recovery
These get your systems revved up for recovery.

MOVEMENT 1:
There are two versions of a twist here. Do one or both.

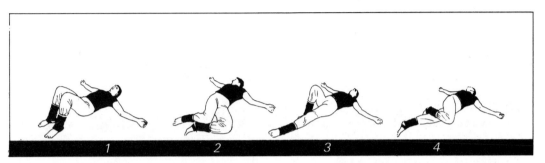

1 Lie on your back with your knees bent. Press your waist onto the floor and keep your feet and knees hip-width apart. Relax your arms out to your sides at shoulder-level and keep your neck relaxed.

2 As you breathe out, roll both knees towards one side of your body. Let them feel very heavy. At the same time, turn your face in the opposite direction to your knees. Hold for two or three breaths then reverse.

3 Roll back to centre and stretch one leg straight out along the floor.

4 As you beathe out, roll your folded leg across your straight leg. At the same time turn your face in the opposite direction of your folded knee. Hold this position for two or three breaths, then roll back to centre and reverse the movement. This twist may be made as large or small as you like, so long as it is painless and comfortable.

Movements for special circumstances

MOVEMENT 2:
The sleeping twist
A gentle twist of the entire spine

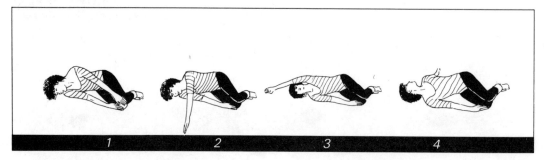

1 Lie on one side in a nearly 'foetal' position. Tuck your knees up close to your body and stretch your arms so that your fingers just touch your knees. Let your head rest over your shoulder onto the floor or a cushion.

2 Keep your lower hand in contact with your lower knee. Begin to circle your upper arm forwards and up over your head. Keep a sense of stretch in your arm and look at your hand as it moves. Your head will need to turn to do this.

3 Continue to circle your arm up over your head. Turn your head to keep your hand in view if you can. Keep your lower hand on your other knee.

4 Circle your arm right round behind you until you touch the back of your pelvis. Look behind you as far as you can. Hold that position for four breaths in and out. Each time you breathe out, let that arm and shoulder feel heavier and more relaxed. Reverse the circle and repeat it on your other side.

TRY THESE TOO:

Movements 4 and 6 from The basic 12 (pages 34 and 35)

Movements 2 and 5 from The top 20 (pages 52 and 54)

Movement 4 from the Posture movements section (page 3)

Movements 1, 2 and 6 from the Articulation movements section (pages 75, 76 and 78)

Movements 1 and 2 from the Breath movements section (pages 90 and 91)

Movements 4 and 8 from the Task-related movements section (pages 97 and 99)

Movements for special circumstances

Trauma, grief and crisis

Some movements have the power to prevent the onset of long-term, deep-seated illness that can result from trauma, grief and crisis. These movements release emotional pain from your body.

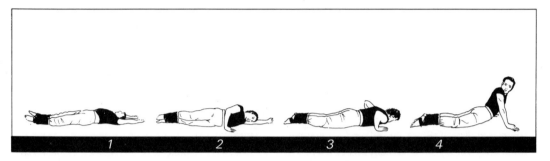

1 Stretch out on the floor with your arms up over your head. Stretch your toes and fingers. Tuck your chin towards your neck. Breathe slowly and deeply.

2 Roll to one side keeping the arm on that side straight. Bring your other arm in front of your chest, palm down. Pause here for another breath.

3 Roll onto your front, folding your straight arm so that both hands rest under your shoulders. Pause here with your forehead lowered. Breathe.

4 Now stretch both arms, or straighten them, so that your head, chest and ribs are lifted. Keep the front of your pelvis pressed onto the floor. Hold this for a few seconds, then turn your head to look over each shoulder. Reverse these sequence of movements until you are resting on your back again. Repeat it if you want to. Be certain to sigh if you feel inclined to.

TRY THESE TOO:

Movements 1, 3, 8, 10 and 12 from The basic 12 (pages 33, 34, 36, 37 and 38)

Movements 4, 12, 13 and 20 from The top 20 (pages 53, 60, 61 and 66)

Movements 4 and 6 from the Articulation movements section (pages 77 and 78)

Movements 5 and 6 from the Stretch movements section (page 81)

Movement 6 from the Balance movements section (page 89)

Movements 1 and 4 from the Breath movements section (pages 90 and 92)

Movements 1, 2, 3 and 7 from the Movements to relieve ailments section (pages 100, 101 and 103)

Afterword

As you see, it is possible for you to include the Movement Design process at many and varied times in your life. Movement Design is based on appropriateness therefore as you or your circumstances changes, so can your practice.

The movements described within this book are yours for a lifetime. You may use them as they are, alter them, speed them up, slow them down, or in any way make them appropriate to you at any one moment in your life.

You may teach them to your children, your mother, your grandfather or your neighbour; you may perform them playfully or seriously; you may practice them daily as a discipline, or somehow include them in your life in a more relaxed manner. However you choose to use them, remember that these movements are simple routes to the personality living within your body. Each is designed to return something to you that really should be yours already. These movements will create changes, they will improve your health and they will invite exuberance back into your life.

And so I must close by wishing you wellness, progress and that very special joyousness that comes through movement.

LET'S COOK IT TOGETHER!

Utterly *SCRUMPTIOUS* Recipes for You and Your Children —— To Make TOGETHER — Vegetarian Style! ——

by
Peggy Brusseau

 KIDS! (Don't let Mum and Dad read this . . .):

Here's a very special cookbook which lets you have all the fun in the kitchen while Mum and Dad help out with the boring bits (who knows, they might even do the washing up!). With just a little help from a grown-up you can make some amazing inventions, such as Stars in a Blizzard, Fruity Goop and Jump and Shout. What are they? Well look inside and you'll be surprised to find they look and taste just as good as they sound. So grab a grown-up and get cooking!

 PARENTS (Kids can skip this bit . . .):

Here's a unique cookery book that is written especially for parents and children to use *together*. All the recipes are quick and easy to make, using healthy, natural ingredients that will teach your children the basics of good food habits quite painlessly. Safety and hygiene in the kitchen are essential aspects which are covered, too. Lots of original, delicious recipes are included, and the clear, step-by-step format divides the tasks between old and young. After all, as the author says: 'The family that cooks together — has a lot of fun together!'